Lasagna *for* Lunch

Declaring Peace with Emotional Eating

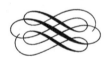

Mary Anne Cohen

New Forge Press

New Forge Press
951 New Forge Road
Ancram, New York 12502

Book designer: Tony Meisel
Printed in the United States of America

ISBN: 978-0-9895656-0-8

Disclaimer
The author and publisher of this book intend for this publication to provide
accurate information. It is sold with the understanding that it is meant to
complement, not substitute for, professional medical and psychological services.
Names and identifying data have been changed for confidentiality.

Dedication

To Michael Scanlon, whose vitality, love, and humor
are vitamins to my soul. Still.

Acknowledgements

To my chosen family, Randy Frankel and Aaron Cohen, Carolyn Marx
Fletcher and Greg Fletcher, Jennifer Scanlon and Bronson Fox, Sean
and Rebecca Scanlon.

To the memory of my cherished parents, Leon and Lily Lifshutz.

Heartfelt appreciation to the women and men who have shared their
life journeys with me. And appreciation for how we learned together to
create the bridge of hope, healing, health, and wholeness.

Special thanks to Laura Shammah, MS, RD for contributing her
expertise on nutrition (chapter 10).

Table of Contents

Acknowledgements   5

Introduction   7

1. Evolving From Impasse to Possibility   14

2. Frozen Grief and Emotional Eating   33

3. The Inner World of the Emotional Eater   54

4. Bodies and Culture: From Combat to Compassion   177

5. Childhood Attachments and Eating Disorders   208

6. The Family: From Conflict to Connection   223

7. Sexual Abuse and Substance Abuse   253

8. From Gridlock to Growth: Confronting Obstacles to Change   283

9. Psychotherapy: A Second Chance   304

10. Food, Glorious Food! Declaring Peace
with Emotional Eating   317

Epilogue. Life after Eating Disorders   343

Introduction

In 1982, I coined the term "emotional eating" to describe the varied and conflicted, fluctuating and frustrating relationship many people have with food.

Emotional eating is when you are lonely in the middle of the night and you look for comfort in the refrigerator.

Emotional eating is when you are angry at someone and you tear and chew into food when you really want to bite that person's head off.

Emotional eating is when you feel bored and empty inside and cannot figure out what to do for yourself, so you binge and make yourself throw up.

Emotional eating is when you refuse to eat and starve yourself because you feel powerless and out-of-control over how your life is going.

Emotional eating is about using food to distract, detour, or deny your inner emotions.

Emotional eating is about being hungry from the heart and not from the stomach.

The women, men, and teenagers I work with battle compulsive overeating, body image dissatisfaction, bulimia, binge eating disorder, anorexia, and chronic dieting. Although people abuse food in many different ways—gorging, bingeing and purging, or starving—all emotional eaters use food as a drug that can soothe, comfort, and keep them company, or even as a weapon to sabotage and hurt themselves.

No matter where they fall on the spectrum—from an 80-pound anorexic to a 450-pound binge-eater—their relationship with food and their bodies is fueled and driven by emotions too hard to digest—sadness and fear, depression, anxiety, grief, trauma, betrayal, anger, sexual problems, feelings of abandonment and rejection.

My first book, *French Toast for Breakfast: Declaring Peace with Emotional Eating* (Gürze Books, 1995; Spanish version, Ediciones Piramide, Madrid, 1997), chronicles my own personal journey through compulsive eating and how I resolved this struggle. Then, in 2008, my mother died. I was suffused with such passionate inner contradictions that food beckoned to me once again. A wild mixture of emotions erupted from within me. I felt deep sadness and yearning for her. At the same time, I felt relief that she was dead. I felt an overwhelming love to her for nurturing the very essence of who I am. And I also felt dark anger for the ways she had hurt me. I wanted her back. I wanted her dead. I believed she would return. I hoped she would. I feared she would. I understood she was dead. I could not understand it was forever.

That same year, another family member lay near death until finally receiving a successful heart transplant. Another loved one had a melanoma removed but then needed open heart surgery. Then another family member developed cancer. And I was still recovering from the death of my father two years before.[1]

My world was crushed. I could not contain all these losses and threats of such frightening proportions. I began to overeat again.

A friend gently counseled me, "Maybe in the midst of all these hard times you could become more conscious every day of the people and blessings that you do have. Maybe this is a time to develop more gratitude and a heightened awareness of what *is* beautiful in your life."

"No way!" I blurted out. "I just want to go back to taking everybody for granted!"

We both burst out laughing. And all my pent-up anxiety and vigilance about who might die next and what upcoming tragedy lurked on the horizon bubbled to the surface. I realized I could not spend the rest of my life fearing when the next shoe would drop and "regretting the future." The absurd notion that I wanted nothing more than to return to a life where I could take everyone for granted injected a note of humor during a bleak time and helped me begin to put things back in perspective.

I realized I needed a lot of quiet time to be with my feelings and listen to myself and digest my experiences. I decided to retreat into emotional intensive care and spend some extended time at my country house in the woods of upstate New York. To be with nature. To unplug from the schedule of everyday life in the city. And to spend time with my husband returning to the natural rhythm of sleeping, waking, walking, reading, cooking, enjoying the sounds of the forest. And visiting with my phoebes.

My phoebe birds, small brown birds with long flicking tail feathers, were already in attendance when I first came to my country house over twenty years ago. They had built a nest over the porch light, and every single year found their way back to that very same porch light from wherever they had migrated during the winter. Every spring they returned to lay eggs and raise new babies. I had no idea what generation we were up to, but I loved their rituals. The mama and papa rimmed the nest with bright green spring moss to soften the home for the babies. After weeks of sitting on the eggs, three little fluffs with beaks would hatch and for the next several weeks, mama and papa would fly back and forth feeding their brood. Finally, the day comes when the first baby stands up in the nest, peers tentatively over the edge, stretches its wings, hops up and down, and takes its first choppy short flight. Mama and papa perch anxiously on a nearby tree, chirping their encouragement.

Witnessing the continuity of the phoebe cycle of life and the inevitability of the babies leaving home and the parents flying away after their job is done filled me with a mixture of sadness, yet also peace and hope about the rhythm of life over which I have no control. And I found a measure of quietude in my heart.

Food returned to just being food. Eating returned to just being eating. My pain returned to being my pain. And my pleasure in life returned to being pleasure.

And then this book got born.[2]

French Toast for Breakfast: Declaring Peace with Emotional Eating is based on the belief that everyone's eating problem is as unique as a fingerprint. I help readers understand the habits, emotions, and addictions that have caused them to resort to bingeing, purging, or starving. And I offer individualized, comprehensive strategies and techniques for declaring peace with emotional eating.

Lasagna for Lunch: Declaring Peace with Emotional Eating chronicles my experiences as an eating disorder therapist for the past forty years. It is an account from behind the scenes of what goes on in private between client and therapist to heal an eating disorder. Learning about the inner workings of the therapist, as well as the inner world of the client, gives a personal view into how the mysterious process of change and recovery evolves.

A person's eating disorder is a creative solution to inner turmoil. The therapist helps expand the creativity of the client to find solutions that are emotionally nurturing, not hurtful. Every patient's needs in therapy are special and personal. The thrust of this book is to explore the ways our relationships with ourselves and others can go awry and lead us to conclude that trusting food is safer than trusting people.

And, finally, I discuss how the relationship with an empathic therapist can help us find the path back to healing, health, and wholeness.

Chapter 1. Evolving from Impasse to Possibility
In this chapter, I share my journey of learning how to decode the heart and soul of eating disorders and how curiosity, self reflection, compassion, and even humor open the door to declaring peace with emotional eating.

Chapter 2. Frozen Grief and Emotional Eating
Loss and unresolved grief can play a significant part in emotional eating. This chapter illustrates how crucial it is for people to mourn the sorrows that have kept them stuck in bingeing, purging, or starving.

Chapter 3. The Inner World of the Emotional Eater
We study the internal landscape of the emotional eater—all the variations on a theme from anorexia to bulimia to binge eating to obesity to men with eating disorders.

Chapter 4. Body Image and Culture
We discuss the conflicts, confusion, and quarrels with our bodies and how to find our way to grow from conflict to contentment.

Chapter 5. Childhood Attachments and Eating Disorders
How did we learn that loving food is safer than loving people? That trusting food is safer than trusting people? We discover how to reclaim a nourishing connection with food, ourselves, and others.

Chapter 6. The Family: From Conflict to Connection
We analyze the family connection—the original cast of characters that may have set the stage for withdrawing into eating problems as a tool to cope with family stress.

Chapter 7. Sexual Abuse and Substance Abuse
The trauma of sexual abuse often impacts emotional eaters. This may lead to substance abuse as well. Recovery involves integrating treatment for both types of abuse.

Chapter 8. From Gridlock to Growth: Confronting Obstacles to Change
We explore motivation, hope, readiness to change and how to overcome the obstacles to discovering your healing path.

Chapter 9. Psychotherapy for Eating Disorders: A Second Chance
The healing relationship between therapist and client provides the bridge between emotional eating and the road to recovery.

Chapter 10. Food, Glorious Food! Declaring Peace with Emotional Eating
What role does food play in your recovery? Come join me in my office for food and nutrition rehabilitation.

A Note About the Title: I am sitting with my dear friend Carolyn in a cozy Italian restaurant on a winter's afternoon. We are getting ready to have one of our delicious heart-to-heart chats. As we read the menu, I think to myself, "I should be good and order a salad. I haven't exercised that much lately, and the salad will be low in calories."

But that's not what I really want. It feels depriving and doesn't match the warmth of the atmosphere and the sharing moment we are about to create. Carolyn, studying her menu, looks up, and we both say simultaneously, "How about lasagna for lunch?!" The rich warmth of the meal with a glass of wine and laughter with my oldest friend sounds just about right!

1 In *The Orphaned Adult: Understanding and Coping with Grief and Change after the Death of Our Parents* (Perseus Publishing, 1999), Alexander Levy describes the particular grief of losing one's second parent and the tumultuous reverberations to one's sense of self.

2 As I watched the phoebes hatch, I realized how much "hatching" is an apt description for the process of healing an eating disorder and giving birth to one's self. Hatching is not an easy task, as one little chick proved as he finally squirmed out of his shell with a tiny hat of shell perched on his head.

Other authors have been intrigued by the metaphor of birds and hatching as well: The naturalist John Burroughs observed, "The live bird is a fellow passenger; we are making the voyage together, and there is a sympathy between us that quickly leads to knowledge."

"Hope" is the thing with feathers— / That perches in the soul— /And sings the tune without the words— / And never stops— at all, wrote Emily Dickinson.

"The key to everything is patience. You get the chicken by hatching the egg, not by smashing it," said psychologist Arnold H. Glasgow.

The poet C.S. Lewis wrote, "It may be hard for an egg to turn into a bird; it would be a jolly sight harder for it to learn to fly while remaining an egg. We are like eggs [but] you cannot go on indefinitely being just an ordinary egg. We must be hatched."

1. Evolving from Impasse to Possibility

Over 40 years ago, when I began training to become a psychotherapist, I wrote down verbatim what my supervisor advised. I memorized it, and then earnestly stated it back to my client. I was so worried about doing the right thing. I depended on my supervisor to tell me what that right thing was.

As time progressed, I mastered the formal expertise of conducting psychotherapy. I grew skilled in the in-depth treatment of eating disorders through psychodynamic, cognitive, and behavioral approaches. I learned how to help clients untangle their personal roadblocks to recovery. I learned when medical evaluation was needed, when medication might be helpful, and when a nutritionist's contribution could support the process.

The Evolution of a Psychotherapist: Behind the Scenes

Only when I became secure and comfortable knowing all these "right" techniques did something shift within me. This was brought home when a colleague, steeped in classical psychoanalysis, discussed with me an incident from her practice. The therapist needed to call a patient to cancel their next appointment because of a funeral the therapist had to attend. When her patient asked with concern, "I'm sorry. Who died?" my colleague refused to disclose that it was her own mother. The patient, in a rage about not being given a straightforward answer, left treatment in a huff.

The therapist believed she was following formal analytic technique which maintains that therapist self-disclosure may "contaminate" the relationship with the patient. But in this case, the analyst had ignored the *human* dimension in therapy when the patient expressed her concern.

My own evolution as a therapist would have led me to say directly, "My mother died." Or, in another situation with a bulimic girl, "When I hear about the abuse you have suffered, it makes me want to throw up too." Or, on other occasions, I have been moved to tears, such as when Frieda cried as she recounted how her grandmother died in a German concentration camp just one day before Liberation. I am no longer afraid to express the full range of my feelings in sessions, when appropriate.

With time and experience, I began to allow my heart and soul to play a larger role in my relationship with my patients.

Foundations of a Fruitful Therapy: The Ground Work
Therapy for emotional eating is not about what you should eat, what you should not eat, how much you should eat, when you should it, and what the calorie count should be. Therapy for emotional eating is about forging a connection between therapist and client that will help illuminate where the person has gotten stuck in his/her emotional life and how this led to seeking "solutions" through bingeing, purging, or starving. Therapy is a joint effort to reweave the torn emotional fabric of the past so the person can live more fully and peacefully in the present.

Psychotherapy is not just about the "reserved and wise" therapist of formal psychoanalysis ministering to the "troubled and needy" patient. Therapy is a collaborative relationship where *trust* between therapist and patient, built over time, is one of the crucial keys that will help unlock and free the patient from the eating disorder. Through this collaboration, genuine change and transformation take place.

Besides trust, other ingredients create a fruitful therapy. The therapist helps the emotional eater recognize that:

- *All behavior has meaning.* There is rhyme and reason to what makes us tick. We often contain many layers and even contradictions within ourselves that need to be understood to heal our problems.
- *A nonjudgmental attitude is vital.* It is hard to get better when we bury ourselves under layers of guilt, shame, and blame.
- *Cultivating curiosity* about what fuels an eating problem as well as other life problems invites a gentle, mindful approach to learning about our self.
- *Self-reflection.* When we are able to step outside of ourselves and observe our own behavior, we are in a stronger position to understand what makes us act in hurtful ways. Self-reflection gives us a new perspective and vantage point which eases the pull to repeat harmful patterns from the past.
- *Verbalizing feelings* lessens the impulse to act on them. Fear, rage, anxiety—all triggers for emotional eating—can be tamed to some degree by verbalizing them which helps let off steam. Words express, describe, and serve as a release valve for intense feelings.
- *Many paths to recovery exist.* There is no "one-right-way" to heal. You and your therapist will uncover your own creative and personal strategies to help you.
- *Resilience* strengthens our ability to cope with pain and stress without resorting to self-defeating behaviors. Resilience is a skill that can be learned.
- *Laughter* lightens the journey. Humor helps the healing. As Mark Twain once said, "Humor is mankind's greatest blessing!"

Curiosity: Kindling New Perspectives

"Do I contradict myself?" Walt Whitman famously asked. "I contain multitudes."

Curiosity, empathy, and a nonjudgmental attitude by the therapist are the vital ingredients that activate a successful therapeutic relationship. Searching to understand the unique meaning in each patient's story provides the key to illuminate how to change hurtful patterns.

A transformative psychotherapy is like Alice in Wonderland peering through the looking glass and remarking with amazement, "Curiouser and curiouser!" Venturing through the looking glass is the perfect image for entering therapy—a journey toward self-reflection and self-discovery.

Over the years, I have treated patients whose issues ranged from relatively mild to very serious. I have chosen some particularly unusual stories from patients to highlight, in a dramatic way, the need for curiosity in therapy. Each has taught me the value of wonderment at the varieties of human experience and demonstrates the remarkable complexity of human nature.

Millie and the "Positive" Meaning of Violence

Millie was shot three times by her jealous boyfriend. Louis was arrested and sent to jail. The doctors retrieved only one of the bullets from her body because of the dangerous position of the other two. Months later, after she recovered, Millie secretly married Louis in jail and told no one. She came to therapy for anxiety, depression, and bulimia. When she confided that she had secretly married the man who shot her, my natural human impulse was to yell, "What the hell is the matter with you? Are you crazy? That man almost killed you!"

Had I responded that way, I would have lost Millie and lost the opportunity to help her. As she sensed my genuine wish to understand her, Millie herself became more curious and self-reflective about why she accepted Louis's behavior. She began to delve deeper, telling me, "My father was a womanizer who abandoned our family when I was five. My father's rejection made me yearn for a man who really cared for me. When Louis shot me in a fit of jealous rage, I believed this proved he truly loved me. The strength of Louis's jealousy has always felt like love." Millie then added with a rueful laugh, "I also realize that with Louis in jail, I will always know where he is on Saturday nights, unlike my poor mother, who never knew where my Dad was!"

In her therapy, Millie came to experience me as someone who cared for her without violence. Our relationship, based on consistent trust as well as curiosity, was new for her. In time, Millie grew more reflective and self-protective. As she became increasingly able to confront the abandonment in her past and its impact on her, she freed herself to make healthier choices. Her bulimia ebbed as her self-assurance grew.

Chelsie and Her Rape Fantasy

Chelsie, a binge eating client, presented a most difficult challenge for me. In one of her therapy sessions, Chelsie described a movie she had seen in which a psychotherapist gets brutally raped. Then she announced calmly, "I wish you were that therapist who got raped."

I was startled and recoiled inwardly at her cruel fantasy. Rather than retaliate with hostility, I summoned up my curiosity. "What would be so good about my being raped? How would that help?" I asked.

Chelsie then revealed she had been raped twice as a teenager. Her wish to see me raped as well was her desperate attempt to compel me to more fully understand her suffering. By injecting into me the traumatic horror she had experienced, Chelsie did succeed in making me viscerally understand how raw and terrified she had felt. In the end, her cruel fantasy deepened our bond and my understanding of her anguish. Connecting more directly with the brunt of her rage and vulnerability helped Chelsie relinquish her binge eating over time.

Greg and the Impact of the Family Secret

Greg, a compulsive overeater, struggled in his relationships with women and his inability to sustain a long-term romance. On her deathbed, Greg's mother confessed that the father Greg had grown up with was not his real father. Greg was born out of wedlock by a different man. To deal with this shocking revelation and to seek help with his overeating, Greg came to treatment.

Greg expressed horror at the betrayal of his mother and stepfather who had kept this secret from him all his life. And yet he also felt a measure of relief and a new clarity, "Certain undercurrents I felt growing up of not belonging and being left out now make sense to me." We devoted our work to understanding how this secret was connected to Greg's mistrustful relationships with the women in his life and his hidden compulsion to overeat. Secrets can keep a person stuck in an eating disorder. Finally revealing them can diminish their impact.

Isabella and How Bigamy "Helped" Her

Isabella suffered from anorexia and was unhappily married. She came to therapy after discovering her husband was also married to another woman. He had children with this other woman and an ongoing relationship with his second family.

Isabella suspected her husband had a secret life for quite some time and began to explore why she denied all the warning signs. Rather than beating herself up about her blindness to the situation, we tried to cultivate her curiosity about why she allowed her "not knowing" to continue and how her anorexia served to numb her feelings and awareness.

Isabella revealed that her father sexually abused her when she was young. The sexual experience with her father instilled guilt in her, making her feel she was to blame for stealing him away from her mother. This guilt from the past left her fearful of having any man exclusively to herself. "Sharing" her husband with his other wife secretly relieved her by limiting the marriage to a part-time relationship. She concluded that having a full-time husband felt too threatening and incestuous. Decoding and appreciating the meaning of her behavior gave Isabella more clarity and freedom to decide what further steps she might want to take regarding her marriage. It also helped her to tackle the necessary self-care to make progress with her anorexia.

Veronica, the Secret Murderer

Veronica came to therapy for a binge eating disorder. She suffered from deep loneliness, had few friends and never had a boyfriend. Veronica disclosed that when she was three years old, her mother had died. Only much later in her therapy did she shamefully "confess" the full truth: "My mother died in childbirth while giving birth to me. I killed her."

Veronica firmly believed she was a murderer. Her shame and guilt caused her to push people away so no one would discover her true "badness"—that she had caused her own mother's death. Confessing this secret helped us better understand the connection between this birth trauma, her conviction about being a toxic person, and her need for the comfort of bingeing. In time, we also understood Veronica's fear that she might kill off anyone she loved just as she believed she had done to her mother.

Ellen versus Elliot

Ellen struggled with a cycle of bingeing and restricting her food. Although Ellen could pass for a woman she was, in fact, a pre-operative transsexual man. Elliot/Ellen was undergoing female hormone injections and hoped one day to have the operation to become a woman. Elliott described how he wanted to become a woman so he could be the lesbian lover of his girlfriend, who also encouraged the surgery. Is this a healthy decision or not? Only curiosity and deepening our understanding of what makes him/her tick will reveal the meaningfulness of this wish. The connection between his gender identity confusion and bingeing (which he related to making him feel rounder and more like a woman) and starving (which made him feel more angular like a man) also needs to be unraveled.

Margaret, Blind to Her Own Body

Margaret, a woman in her early 30s with a binge eating disorder, spoke of how her social isolation and loneliness often prompted her to overeat. She also admitted she had never looked at her own body naked. She claimed to have never seen herself without clothes in a full-length mirror. She never looked down while showering and never had a sexual relationship. During her short time in therapy, Margaret, a bright and sensitive woman, could not remember any significant history or experience to explain her dread of looking at her own body.

Although we searched for the meaning of her unusual body phobia, we never discovered it. However, in our discussions about her life and feelings, Margaret felt accepted and understood. She came from a large family that gave her little attention; she felt "unseen" by her parents. Just being listened to and valued was a new experience for her. Shortly into her therapy, Margaret met a man whom she grew to trust and love. She had sex for the first time, they married, and she felt happy and at ease. Although we never unraveled her mystery, Margaret managed to overcome inner barriers that had blocked her from forming an intimate relationship. Years later, Margaret wrote to me expressing her enjoyment of her life and her increased freedom from binge eating.

Beatrice and Her Full-Time Underground Secret

Beatrice has kept her bulimia of 35 years a complete secret from her husband, despite being married for 25 years. Why does she need to keep this hidden? Why is she so afraid of being found out? What does it mean to reveal and share and confide in her husband? These are the questions I hope Beatrice will become curious about.

Kristen, a Serial Abortion Seeker

Kristen, a physician's assistant with an extensive medical background, allowed herself to become pregnant seven times and had seven abortions. She also had a significant history of bulimia. Why would an educated woman with medical knowledge and resources allow this to happen repeatedly? How does her "bingeing and purging" on pregnancies relate to her bulimia? We need to encourage Kristen's curiosity so we may uncover the meaning of her compulsive pattern and protect her from future risky behavior.

Abuse, Betrayal, Religion, and Eating Disorders

Yvonne and Felicia, two binge eaters, were both molested by their fathers, both ministers. Becky, also a binge eater, was beaten frequently by her father, a rabbi, who then expected Becky to kiss his hand after he hit her. He wanted her to express gratitude that she had a father who was trying to raise her properly.

What is the impact of these untrustworthy religious fathers on their daughters' eating disorders? All three girls need to seek out why bingeing became their attempt to stuff down their rage, powerlessness, and fear—a pattern they carried into adult life.

Fostering Resilience: Moving from Gridlock to Growth

And then the day came, when the risk to remain tight in a bud
was more painful than the risk it took to blossom.
—Anaïs Nin

We tend to think of resilience as an inborn mechanism that makes some people better at handling stress and bouncing back from hurtful or traumatic experiences. We say someone is "a tough hombre" or "she's a tough cookie" or "he can really roll with the punches."

Temperamentally, some babies are born more spunky than others.

Some are more sensitive; some are more confident, some are more vulnerable. Parents can strengthen their child's resilience by providing them with "roots and wings," the roots of deeply grounded security and the wings to eventually separate, be unique, and soar.

The case of Deirdre illustrates her inherent resilience in handling a traumatic situation. Deirdre, struggling with obesity and a binge eating disorder, is a 40-year-old woman who grew up in a home with ongoing violence. Her parents were volatile but, thankfully, she had a devoted grandmother; many of her teachers were fond and supportive of her. This helped build the cornerstones of her resilience.

Deirdre described a most poignant and amazing example of resilience. One afternoon when she was six, she was playing in her room and heard her parents fighting. Rushing out to the living room, she witnessed her father choking her mother. Deirdre's mother screamed to her, "Get a knife from the kitchen! Stab him! He's killing me!" Deirdre was terrified, wanting to protect and obey her mother on one hand, but certainly not wanting to stab or injure her father on the other. Not knowing what to do, she ran into the kitchen in a panic and discovered a small plastic fork from a take-out restaurant. She began poking her father in the back with this little plastic fork. Irritated by the jabbing of the plastic utensil, he let go of Deirdre's mother. Through her amazing natural resilience, Deirdre saved the day. Her creative solution protected both her mother and her father and protected her relationship with each of them as well.

Although Deirdre developed a binge eating disorder and went on to marry a violent man who beat her, she eventually was able to reverse the family pattern through her therapy.[1] Through self-reflection, the yearning to break the painful family chains that bound her, and the development of a loving attachment with her therapist, Deirdre came to believe she could create a different road map for her life. She remarried a kind, gentle man who had triumphed over adversity through his own resourcefulness. They became devoted parents, and she is a successful professional helping foster children. Deirdre's early resilience became strengthened in therapy which enabled her to apply new found coping strategies to overcome her eating disorder.

The psychologist Tian Dayton writes, "Resilient people do have emotional and psychological scars that they carry from their experience. They indeed struggle, but they keep going. *Resilience is not the ability to escape unharmed. It is the ability to thrive in spite of the odds.*"[2]

The Giorgios illustrate an example of family resilience. The Giorgios, immigrants recently arrived in America, desperately wanted to celebrate a beautiful Christmas in their new land, but had no money to spare. The family concluded they would wait until after Christmas, when other families were throwing out their Christmas trees on the curb. They then went "shopping" to collect a discarded tree, brought it home, and created their own delayed holiday. Their resourceful inventiveness triumphed over their deprivation. This was truly thinking outside the box!

The skills of resilience can be developed and become an important tool to heal an eating disorder. Strengthening our psychological "grit" provides alternatives to emotional eating. It is a process over time, just like building strong muscles.

It can be delightful to watch a little child learn to unapologetically identify and claim her needs, the foundation of resilience. Sasha, a secure, expressive two-year-old, has added two new words to her vocabulary: "More" and "All done." She will let you know in no uncertain terms when she wants more food *and* when she's all done. When she wants to play some more *and* when she's had enough. When she wants more cuddles *and* when she's all done and ready to climb off your lap.

The emotional eater, on the other hand, has lost that capacity of self-regulation and instead recruits food to remedy a host of problematic issues that have nothing to do with hunger and fullness. For the anorexic, the most fluent expression is "all done." For the overeater, the constant word is "more." And the bulimic wants "more and all done" both at the same time as she gorges and purges her food in one fell swoop.

Fostering resilience begins with discovering the "Power of One." Focusing on one step at a time, we begin with "bite-size pieces" to strengthen our strategies against emotional eating. The Power of One teaches us:

- To take ONE second, minute, or day at a time.
- To set ONE goal at a time.
- To deal with ONE problem at a time.
- To eat ONE more bite or meal than you are prepared for if you are anorexic.
- To resist ONE more binge episode.
- To reduce your number of purge episodes by ONE more.
- To make ONE more healthy choice.
- To find ONE more thing you appreciate about your body.
- To take ONE more breath to calm yourself down.
- To continue to put ONE foot in front of the other, even when you feel discouraged.
- To trust your body and treat it right for ONE more day.
- To identify and process ONE more emotion at a time.[3]

Resilience has been called "ordinary magic."[4] You can cultivate further strategies to build your ordinary magic by:

Lessening your perfectionism. The identity of many emotional eaters is based on performance, pleasing, and striving to be perfect; they are convinced this is what makes them lovable. However, evaluating your life and your eating behavior through the lens of "I must be perfect" will sign you on for a lifetime of frustration and self-doubt. Most often, "good enough is good enough."

Erin lamented she was no longer a size zero, "my ideal size." I had known Erin at size 0, a gaunt young woman with angular collar bones that jutted out alarmingly. She was scary-looking then. Erin caught herself midstream in being self-critical and relented, "OK, I guess after three children, I have to learn to be more realistic. I'm allowed to be a larger size with a little tummy to show for all my hard work of carrying three kids. My perfectionism could lead me straight back to anorexia. I need to remember it was my learning *healthy* eating that allowed me to get pregnant in the first place."

Talking to yourself and being your own guidance counselor. Tony groans, "Today was a horrible day with my boss. I now know I have a choice to binge and throw up to make myself feel better in the moment. Or I can distract myself until that mood passes and have a healthy carrot juice instead. I'll feel a hell of a lot better tomorrow for not giving in."

Complaining, crying, even howling, and not bottling up hurtful feelings can be a satisfying way of expressing oneself that does not involve detouring emotions through eating behaviors. By developing a variety of techniques of self-expression, emotional eating does not have to be the only game in town. The comedian Lily Tomlin once declared, "God gave humans the gift of language, so we could complain!" And sometimes using your mouth for "purging" frustration in words and not using it for overeating brings satisfaction from tension and relief.

Estee, an anorexic and bulimic patient who was taught all her life to "suck it up," enjoyed my giving her permission to complain. She enjoyed this new found freedom so much that she bought me a coffee mug with this scene on it: A man goes to the Complaint Department of a store and is asked by the clerk what his grievance is. The customer replies, "Pretty much everything!"

Talking to others who have the ability to just listen (and not necessarily give advice). Venting our stress rather than acting out with food is a robust tool to lighten our burden. "I love coming to therapy," laughed Shelley, "because you have to fully listen to me and I don't have to reciprocate by being polite and asking how you're doing! Frankly, I don't care how you are. I just want to talk about myself!"

Tolerating feelings. Although they can be very intense, feelings are not facts. Thoughts are not facts. Sometimes, in the heat of the moment, we distort how bad things really are. Bad feelings will pass whether or not we binge, starve, or throw up. Tolerating, expressing, and digesting challenging feelings, rather than acting destructively, builds resilience muscles for the next time a wave of strong emotions threatens to overtake us.

Changing what you can, accepting what you can't. Accept a certain amount of powerless. Take all necessary steps to fix a problem, let go of the results. In the midst of a grueling divorce, Pearl recognized that all the cake in the world was not going to resolve her conflict. She continued her plan of action to solve the legal dilemma while working valiantly not to compound her own pain by overeating.

Meditate on your breathing. Visualize what you need, ask the universe for peace of mind, and give gratitude for what you do have.

Practice self-care. These self-care rituals provide balance and inner harmony: enjoyable exercise, nutritious abundant food, deep sleep, relaxation, good sex, and times of peace and quiet to recharge your batteries.

Find perspective. Tian Dayton writes, "Resilient people tend not to let adversity define them. They see their problems as temporary rather than a permanent state of affairs and tend not to globalize. They find reasons and ways—whether religious, creative, or good common sense—to place a temporary framework and perspective around the problems in their lives."[5]

Everyone's path to self-care and self-soothing is as unique as a fingerprint. Keep refining your unique path. The last chapter has not yet been written on your life. There is still room and time to cultivate a good, strong relationship with yourself where food is no longer a tool for emotional expression and release.

The Healing Power of Laughter

At the height of laughter, the universe is flung into a
kaleidoscope of new possibilities.

—Jean Houston, Ph.D.

Exploring one's inner feelings can be a painful challenge, but humor eases and supports the journey, providing a lighthearted perspective. Sometimes laughter is the best medicine. Where there is humor, there is hope.

Laughter is one of the best devices to handle stress. To laugh at our quirks provides relief, a temporary escape from ourselves, and a reprieve from our problems.

I believe that therapist and client laughing together in the therapy session provides a shared moment of affection and bonding. Therapy is not all hard work, grit, and determination. Humor offers moments of playful connection and a sense of partnership; it is the antidote to the perfection, rigidity, and depression so often experienced by eating-disordered people.

Amber, struggling with severe bulimia, had long expressed a fascination with vampires. We discussed how she identified with the insatiability of the vampire and how when she binged her "fangs" came out. In one of her sessions, Amber described the latest vampire romance novel she was reading. Caught up in the story, I asked Amber, "So what finally happened to this vampire couple?"

A mischievous smile crossed her face and Amber replied, "They lived *capillary* ever after!" We laughed uproariously. Amber had added a most playful note to a very tough struggle. This moment of shared laughter declared, "We're in this together, we are a team, and we'll fight this bulimia together!"

Tyler, an anorexic young man, was describing the impact of his father's death on his eating struggles. "And how did your Dad die?" I asked.

Tyler answered with a rueful half smile, "My father was an alcoholic. He died of *neurosis* of the liver!" In the midst of a sorrowful time, Tyler had found a shred of playfulness that lightened his grief and brought us together on our journey.

Molly, a binge eater, poked fun at herself, "The most stable men in my life have always been Ben and Jerry!" I responded that one of my best girlfriends used to be Sara Lee. We joined together with an affectionate, laughing connection.

"You're the same old boring therapist always trying to psychoanalyze me," complains Trudy, not wanting to speak further about a topic I'm encouraging her to discuss. Knowing Trudy for a long time, I reply, "And you're the same old boring resistant patient always trying to make me feel like a pain-in-the-neck shrink." We both laugh, let off steam at how we are annoying each other, clear the air, and then go back to business.

Geneen is dismayed by her husband's constant criticisms and her own pattern of bingeing every time she feels powerless to confront him. We are working on strengthening her ability to stand up to him. She does not yet feel ready to dish out her words to him, but wants to learn to claim her own power. "Since you're not ready yet to say anything directly to George," I suggest, "why not just practice rolling your eyes, at least in private? Rolling your eyes is a great way to vent some hostility and maybe prevent a binge!" Geneen tentatively rolled her eyes, "Like this?" she asked. "No, like this," I exaggeratedly rolled my eyes. We laughingly began playing at who could roll their eyes more dramatically. She called this our "eye-rolling event." Although this was not an ultimate solution to her conflict with her husband, nor an end to all her binge eating, she enjoyed the playfulness of discovering an alternative to either silence or overeating as she continued to find her own solutions.

Amelia, an Hispanic compulsive overeater, described her childhood in which her mother forced her to clean their apartment every day. Amelia was not allowed to go out and play unless she first scoured the house, which was never quite clean enough for her mother's approval. Reflecting on her mother's obsession with cleanliness, Amelia laughed, although with some regret, "We may have been 'spics,' but at least we were Spic 'n Span!"

We can laugh together because Amelia knows I am an aficionada of all things Hispanic. She feels free to make this gibe with me.

Vivian, a bulimic woman, describes her enjoyment of sexual bondage with ropes. Although she has made some connection between her bulimia and bondage, she is uncertain how much more detail she wants to disclose to me. Unaware of what I am saying, I comment, "By not discussing this further, *you are tying my hands* as I try to understand you better." Vivian looks at me in astonishment, I catch my Freudian slip, and we begin to laugh heartily. This smoothes the way for further communication.

Sometimes eating disorder clients will mention a favorite joke. Often the joke is about food and eating and gives us an insight into their particular conflicts. As a young girl, my favorite joke involved a mother cannibal who is cooking up a captured hostage in a big cauldron in the jungle. Her little cannibal son is poking the man with a fork. The mother scolds the boy, "How many times have I told you not to play with your food!"

Only years later did I consider the possible connection between my enjoyment of this joke and my own compulsive eating. I realized I felt sorry for the young cannibal whose eating was criticized by his mother, since my own eating was often criticized by my mother. But I was also gleeful that the cannibal boy was getting scolded by his mother, because it made me feel I wasn't the only one! On a more subtle level, the joke also helped me feel superior to the boy, since I was pretty sure my cravings to binge would never get to the point of wanting to eat a boiled man out of a cauldron in the jungle.

Laughter is a form of "non-food nurturance," a way of soothing oneself rather than bingeing, starving, or throwing up. Norman

Cousins once declared, "Laughter is inner jogging." Charlie Chaplin once said, "To truly laugh, you must be able to take your pain and play with it."

"There is a great value in humor because it can to some degree positively alter our emotional states when we are faced with cruel reality. Humor is the emotionally healthy way of dealing with the problems and dilemmas of life, as opposed to unhealthy ways such as drug addiction, depression . . . The ability to use humor easily is a wonderful psychological aid . . . Laughter is an appropriate way for the therapist to express his own humanity to the patient."[6]

All the formal therapy techniques in the world are not sufficient to help someone relinquish their pain and their eating disorder. But when the person experiences the therapist as an emotional companion on the journey toward healing, then the process becomes vivid and alive. The root of the word "companion" derives from Latin and means "to break bread." (com = with, pan = bread). To break bread is an act of sharing, of togetherness, of comfort, of being present in the moment—the recipe for a wonderful therapy.[7]

Fortified with curiosity, empathy, resilience, and humor, let's continue our journey to declare peace with emotional eating.

1 The root of the word "family" and "familiar" are the same. We tend to repeat our family patterns—both the loving and the painful ones—simply because they are familiar. What is familiar feels safe, while change can feel dangerous. Unless we identify the chains from the past, we will not be able to untangle the molds we want to break.

2 Tian Dayton, *Emotional Sobriety* (Health Communications, 2008), 103. Emphasis added.

3 Adapted from Tamara Richardson, Ph.D., "The Power of One," www.eatingdisordersrecoverytoday.com/print/nl_edt_15print.html.

4 A.S. Masten, "Ordinary Magic: Resilience Processes in Development," *American Psychologist*, 2001, vol. 56, 227–238; http://psycnet.apa.org/journals/amp/56/3/227.pdf.

5 Tian Dayton, *Emotional Sobriety*, 101.

6 Louis Birner, "Humor and the Joke in Psychoanalysis," in Herb Strean, ed., *The Use of Humor in Psychotherapy* (Jason Aronson, 1994), 81,87.

7 In discussing the death of his wife, Enrique reached for a tissue to wipe his tears. And, surprisingly, he handed me a tissue as well. Although I was not crying, I understood his gesture to mean he wanted a partner to join him in his sorrow. He did not want to cry alone.

2. Frozen Grief and Emotional Eating

Suppressed grief suffocates,
it rages within the breast,
and is forced to multiply its strength.

—Ovid

Patty was an obese binge eater who came to therapy prompted by a diagnosis of pre-diabetes. We began to discuss what triggered her history of overeating and about her life experiences. In a most casual way, she mentioned the early death of her father.

Patty was four years old when her father died. He had been sick for several years and when he died, her family told her, "Daddy went to Heaven. He is in a better place." Daddy was never spoken about again.

"Tell me about him," I asked. "There's nothing to tell," Patty replied. And with that, she began to cry as the accumulation of 32 years of stifled tears came surging up in a tidal wave of pain.

"Oh my God. I have never shed tears for my father before," Patty sobbed.

With each following session, Patty cried deeply about the death of her father. Then one day she exclaimed, "I wonder if after so many years my fat has been like frozen grief. I think with all these tears, my grief is becoming liquid!"

Grief—frozen by fat, frozen by the numbing of overeating, starving, or purging—can be held in the body for years and even decades.

Patty's description of "frozen grief" reminded me of a special moment I spent with my grandmother many years ago. Grandma was 86 at the time and was telling me about her father who had died when she was only five years old. To my astonishment, Grandma began to cry about her father's death—a memory from 81 years before. In that moment, I learned that grief has no timetable. Time does not necessarily heal all wounds. Unspoken loss continues to exert its power. There is no expiration date to memories or pain.

I came to see how much loss and grief can play a significant part in the emotional eating of my patients. I thought about how chronic eating disorders can be related to unresolved frozen grief. And I came to see how therapy for emotional eating needs to help people mourn the sorrows that have kept them stuck in bingeing, purging, or starving.

I began asking my patients to construct a list of losses they had suffered in their lives. I discovered that these losses did not always have to do with death, but with a myriad of ways that hurt can lodge inside us without resolution. Unable to dislodge the "knot" in their throat by crying and grieving, many eating disorder patients turn to bingeing, purging, or starving.

Louise, bulimic and anorexic, described her losses and pain: "I came from a poor family where neither of my parents was able to hold down full-time work. We had to move all the time during my childhood because we couldn't pay the rent. No sooner did I try to make friends at school, then we had to abruptly leave the neighborhood.

I eventually married and found out my husband was having an affair with my best friend. After we divorced, he then married her. I went through two losses for the price of one."

To look at Louise, you would never know she harbored so many traumatic ruptures. Although she was highly intelligent with a close circle of girlfriends, the unspoken, underground fears and anguish of her early life continued to exert their pull. They led her to seek the pain-relieving medication of purging and starving. Unable to connect with the rage at her lifelong deprivation, Louise could not move forward to mourn.

Only when Louise took the time in her therapy to untangle and express her anger and vulnerability could she allow me (and herself) to empathize with the inner little girl who was not well taken care of. Nurtured by our relationship, she finally began to mourn her sorrows which helped her restore healthier eating.

Walter came from a wealthy family with houses, a boat, maids, and nannies. He was bulimic since his early teens and, in spite of the family's wealth, had his own list of hardships that he had never discussed or sorted through—the opposite spectrum from Louise. He revealed: "I knew early on that my mother was cheating on my father—she had a woman lover. My mother ferried me around to our various homes, and she had a parade of different nannies taking care of me and my brother.

"Both of my parents were heavy drinkers and completely self-involved. My father died of alcoholism when I was 20."

Walter had suffered ongoing neglect from both parents, ruptures with homes and nannies, and the traumatic death of his father. "Bulimia is an all-consuming compulsion which has helped me ignore my hurt. When I'm not eating and purging, I'm very depressed. I'd rather be eating and purging."

Mourning for what he did not have, for what he wished he had, and for what he never would have was bitterly painful for Walter. His bulimia provided a cocoon of deadness. With time, and with therapy plus a support group, he became less detached from his feelings and was filled with great anger and sadness.

Feeling bad was actually progress for Walter. He was finally feeling rather than numbing. As he absorbed the ongoing companionship and compassion from his therapist and support group, the warmth of these connections helped him speak about his painful experiences and thaw his grief. The comfort of other people enabled him to relinquish the protection of bulimia and embrace new possibilities of trusting and supportive relationships.

Blanca alternated between binge eating and chronic dieting: "I never had any big trauma in my life, just drama. I had this constant grinding fear and unhappiness, with my parents always yelling, screaming, fighting. The atmosphere in our house—at the dinner table, even on vacation—was fraught with tension and upset. I knew my parents didn't love each other. It always hurt like hell, but when I discovered dieting and overeating, I just froze, and the pain didn't matter so much anymore."

Maureen, a binge eater, described an example of her grandmother's frozen grief. The grandmother's favorite child, her only son, a beautiful boy with bright red hair, died when he was two years old. Several years later, the grandmother had a little daughter—Maureen's mother. When this little daughter turned two years old, the grandmother began dying her hair a bright red as if attempting to resurrect her son. Frozen grief. There is no passage of time.

What Is Grief?

Grief is the normal and natural emotional reaction to any kind of loss. The symptoms of grief are varied:

Anger
Guilt
Crying
Loneliness
Emptiness
Depression
Anxiety

Insomnia/oversleeping

Missing, yearning, longing

Remembering, reviewing

Despair

Feeling like you are going crazy and losing your mind

Bingeing, purging, starving, rigid dieting

Mourning is the process of sorting out these emotions. We experience, explore, express, and integrate our grief, finally adjusting to going on with our lives despite our loss. It is the inner process of letting go.

Mourning is not a linear progression of moving from point A to point Z and then we are done. Mourning does not have a distinct beginning, middle, and end. Rather, it is like being lost at sea. Some memories and emotions, like strong ocean waves, knock you down by their sheer force. Other waves are gentle, lapping at your feet, making you smile with a soft sadness. Mourning has its ebbs and flows—a high tide with upsurges and hidden riptides that can ambush you and flood you with heartache. And mourning has a low and placid tide. Everyone's grief and mourning are profoundly personal.

Other Losses

Death is not the only grief that wounds our heart and soul. Any loss or change or trauma or transition in our lives can feel like a threat to our sense of stability and self.

One of the most unusual experiences of grief I have witnessed was that of Rodolfo, a family friend who had suffered through the earthquake in Mexico City of 1985, which killed 10,000 people. Although Rodolfo did not lose any loved ones, he became quite depressed, "Because of this earthquake, I no longer trust gravity—something you just always take for granted. I trusted gravity and it betrayed me and my country. I feel like I've lost my innocence and faith in the universe." Rodolfo literally had the "earth pulled out from under him" and was grieving this trauma.

Many kinds of loss can trigger significant grief:

Divorce
Marital separation
Breakup of romantic relationship
Personal injury or illness
Family injury or illness
Losing one's job/home
Retirement
Financial loss
Suicide in the family (which also causes shame, secrecy, and feelings of betrayal)
Sexual or physical abuse/violence
Family member serving in the military
Miscarriage/abortion/fertility problems
Menopause
Giving up driving because of age or health
Death of a beloved pet
National tragedy, such as 9/11 or hurricanes Katrina and Sandy
Anticipatory grief: When we know that someone we care for is going to die, we begin the emotional rehearsal for the upcoming loss
Stopping smoking/drinking/drugging/eating disorder behaviors

We suffer losses not only through death. As Judith Viorst writes, we feel loss "also by leaving and being left, by changing and letting go and moving on. And our losses include not only our separations and departures from those we love, but our losses of romantic dreams, impossible expectations, illusions of freedom and power, illusions of safety—and the loss of our own younger self, the self that thought it always would be unwrinkled and invulnerable and immortal."[1]

Why Do Emotional Eaters Freeze Grief?

Our culture, deeply uncomfortable with death, dying, and grieving, encourages us to stifle our feelings. Mourners are advised:

> God never gives you more than you can handle.
> Keep busy!
> Be strong!
> Just give it time.
> Time heals all wounds.
> He's in a better place.
> You need to snap out of your isolation and start getting out more.
> Keep a stiff upper lip. (I imagine that "keeping a stiff upper lip" is a person's attempt to quiet the "trembling lower lip.")

Frozen grief can best be described as grief on hold, partial grief, suppressed grief, complicated mourning, survivor guilt, and unfinished business. Sometimes, absence makes the heart grow *frozen*.

Emotional eaters, obviously, are not the only people to freeze grief. But emotional eaters are prone to derail, detour, and divert difficult feelings through food. And grief is the most difficult of feelings!

Emotional eaters believe if they open their hearts to feel their pain, it will never end. "If I ever started to cry, I would never be able to stop," Yvette, an anorexic woman, declared. Simon, a bulimic man, stated, "My Dad has been dead two months already. I should be over it already and shouldn't really feel sad anymore."

Yvette and Simon's beliefs about grief reveal common traits of people with eating disorders: impatience with themselves, the conviction that strong feelings are scary and should be avoided, black or white thinking, and critical and perfectionist commandments to the self. Emotional eaters prefer a "quick fix" rather than tolerating the process of digesting either food or feelings. No wonder they turn to the numbing and anesthetizing substance of food in an attempt to cover up their sorrow and anger and "just get over it."

But grief *is* painful, it is supposed to be! Grieving is the process of untangling the loss of emotional connections to people or experiences that have great meaning to us. And that hurts.[2]

When someone dies, our mourning freezes if we narrowly view the person as either all good or all bad. This is especially true for eating disorder sufferers who tend to see the world in black and white. (I lost two pounds = I'm good. I gained two pounds = I'm bad.) They are often likely to see their dead loved one as either good or bad, a saint or a sinner. When we cannot accept that most relationships are a mixture of the good with the bad, we get stuck and derailed in the process of mourning. Grief freezes as we commit to viewing this person from just one perspective, without nuances.

Sergio, a classmate, invited me to his house for lunch many years ago. I knew he lived with his brother and that their mother had died seven years before. I was astonished to see that his mother's bedroom appeared untouched from the day she died. In the center of her bed was her nightgown and an old-fashioned black patent leather pocketbook. It lay open, as if waiting for the mother to pack up her powder puff and go out shopping. The brothers had also taken to propagating rubber plants, hundreds of them throughout the house, in every corner and window. It felt like a shrine of sorts to their dead mother, and it felt like years had frozen in this mausoleum, preserving their dead mother and the brothers from the passage of time.

Sergio described his mother as a saint who had never done any wrong. Yet Sergio's life was stultified—he had no social life, no friends, no girlfriend. Just his brother, his mother's pocketbook, and the rubber plants. He could not progress in his mourning because he feared facing the pain of saying goodbye forever or, perhaps, becoming aware of her less than perfect attributes. Instead, he clung to her perfection but at the price of stunting his growth and development.

An opposite example of frozen grief was the case of Marlena. In her mind, her dead mother was the sinner of the century. Unable to find a shred of daughterly love for her mother, Marlena refused to attend her mother's funeral. Although her mother had, indeed, been a difficult and critical person, she could also be loving, generous, and creative. She wasn't just one way. When Marlena finally installed her mother's gravestone, it was shocking in its bare bones approach. It read: "Wife, Mother, Grandmother." She was unable to find in her heart one small adjective to favorably describe her mother. I think it may be the only headstone in the world without a warm or loving word in its description.

How would Marlena's refusal to honor her mother's life be considered frozen grief? When we commit to an ideal image of a mother, as Sergio did, or an all-diabolic view like Marlena's, we freeze ourselves from making peace in our hearts. Sergio, with a falsely exalted view of his mother, stayed stuck in the past. Marlena, filled with resentment and bitterness, never really buried her mother emotionally, but instead carries her around like a stone in her heart.

Hope Edelman, age 13 when her mother died, writes poignantly in *Motherless Daughters: The Legacy of Loss* about the need to embrace ambivalent feelings in order to complete our mourning: "To mourn a mother fully we have to look back at the flip sides of perfection and love. Without this, we remember our mothers as only half of what they were."[3]

I personally resonate with this ambivalent range of emotions in living with, loving, and finally letting go of my mother. My husband and I are going to visit my mother in the assisted living facility where she lived for the last two years of her life. My husband pleads with me while driving there, "Can you really try this time not to wind up screaming at your mother? Just this once."

"Absolutely," I answer, not understanding why he feels compelled to ask. Screaming at my mother is not something I believe I do. After all, I am the dutiful and loving daughter going to visit her mother. But 15 minutes after arriving, I am exceedingly irritated by my mother's commandments, her criticisms, and her controlling. I'm shrieking loudly at her. I cannot contain myself.

And yet, after I scream my head off and we come to some sort of peace, the visit starts winding down. Always in the same way. She is sitting in her recliner chair by the window of her room at the assisted living home. I get down on my knees and put my head in her lap. She runs her tiny gnarled and arthritic fingers through my hair, "My beautiful daughter," she murmurs, "my beautiful daughter."

"Mama, Mama," I whisper into her lap. I cannot believe she is really going to leave me. Forever.

Grieving thaws and mourning progresses when we can realistically perceive the good, the bad, and the indifferent of the person who has left us. Most people are a mingling of loving and flawed, wonderful and hurtful, kind and sometimes mean. Only when mourners are able to acknowledge the full range of attributes in the person they have lost can they integrate their memories in a way that will lead to genuine healing.

A line from Thornton Wilder's *The Bridge of San Luis Rey* describes the hopeful grace of productive mourning, "There is a land of the living and a land of the dead and the bridge is love, the only survival, the only meaning."[4]

Unfreezing Grief: Restarting the Process of Mourning

No pain is so devastating as the pain a person refuses to face . . .
—Glenn Schiraldi[5]

When we are in pain, we naturally seek to protect ourselves from the hurt. And so, after a deep loss, people often sleep, drink, eat, shop, lose themselves on the computer, or engage in any number of activities to dull the ache and fill up the empty space within. But when eating disorders or other addictions become an *ongoing* pattern and a way to *chronically* avoid pain, then grief becomes frozen. The substances quell the pain from the outside in. Real and lasting relief comes from unraveling our emotions from the inside out.

However, we cannot selectively numb only painful memories without also tamping down happy memories as well. The energy used to suppress painful feelings also suppresses all feelings. So, when mourning is on hold, our life is on hold.

Healing grief does not mean you have forgotten the person or thing you lost. It means that the grief finds a place to live in your heart where you are enriched by loving memories and not tormented by anguished ones.

Sometimes grief never gets resolved. Hope Edelman speaks of the Resolution Hoax: "I wish I believed that mourning ends one day or that grief disappears for good. The word resolution dangles before us like a piñata filled with promise, telling us we only need to approach it from the right angle to obtain its prize. Some losses you truly don't get over. Grief is something that continues to get reworked."[6]

We are a group of 40 New Yorkers sitting on an outdoor terrace having lunch at the Hotel Nacional in Havana, Cuba. We are giddy with the freedom of having escaped New York's latest December snowstorm to revel in this warm, tropical paradise. We are enjoying our mojitos and our arroz con pollo as we listen to the music of the Buena Vista Social Club.

Hannah, one of the women in our group, begins to speak, "Twenty years ago, my husband and I were driving our daughters to college in Boston. We pulled off the highway onto the grass because our car was overheating. We all got out of the car to wait for the car to cool down when a truck veered into us. My husband and my daughters were killed instantly."

This moment freezes in time as we all fall silent. We don't know what to say.

Over the years I have thought about the meaning and the timing of Hannah's declaration.

It could mean:

- I have gone on with my life as proven by this exotic trip to Cuba. But in the midst of my pleasure, I would like to take a moment to pay tribute to my dead family. If only they could be here with me. May they rest in peace.
- Every enjoyable experience I have gets ruined by my intrusive memories of the family I have lost. I just have to blurt it out.
- I feel safe in this group of people and would like to share the most intimate wound in my heart.
- Why should you all be enjoying this day while I am still grieving? I want to puncture the happiness of this group. Since pleasure invariably gets spoiled for me, let me spoil it for others as well.

Maybe Hannah's grief contains all these elements. Her life does go on. Her trauma lives on as well.

Grieving is ambiguous. It concludes, it continues, it intrudes, it retreats, it pounces, it ebbs, it flares up, it settles down. Perhaps, like Hannah, we need to learn to contain within us the contradiction that life does go on, there are still pleasures to be enjoyed, and yet we are forever altered by having lost and suffered.

The Process of Thawing Grief

The first step of thawing grief is to tell the story of your loss to safe and empathic people you trust. Sorrow needs to speak. As Shakespeare wrote: "Give sorrow words; the grief that does not speak / Whispers the o'er fraught heart, and bids it break."

Thawing grief includes:

Recounting the story of what happened:

"I was raped on my college campus."

"My boyfriend, Jimmy, was killed in a motorcycle accident."

"My grandmother died of cancer in our house when I was twelve."

Describing the impact it had on you when it occurred:

"The rape devastated me because I had never been with a man before. I feel ruined."

"Jimmy and I were planning to get engaged in June. I will never get married now."

"Watching my grandmother grow increasingly sick frightened me beyond what I could bear. She was ugly, and I didn't know her anymore."

Express the feelings of anger/guilt/self blame/regrets you may have:

"I never should have been walking alone at night on campus. The rape was my fault. But, on the other hand, shouldn't I have the freedom to walk by myself without having to worry I'd get assaulted? I am furious with God for letting this happen to me."

"If only I had reminded Jimmy how wet the roads were that night. But he was always a reckless driver, in my opinion, and I am angry that he may have brought this on himself."

"I feel like a bad person because I wanted my grandmother to die. It was too much for me to handle anymore."

Imagine the effect this loss will have on your life as you move forward:

"I have no idea how I will ever have sex, even with someone I trust. Sex equals trauma in my mind. How will I ever get over this?"

"Will I ever fall in love again? My world has been shattered, and I don't know if I'm ever going to recover."

"If anyone knew the real me—that I wanted Grandma to finally die—they would never look at me the same way again."

Consider the connection between your loss and your history of bingeing, purging, starving, drinking, taking drugs, or any other addictions.

Allow yourself to feel the physical impact of your story.
Do you want to eat, drink, run away, or cry? Crying is our natural healing process of releasing emotions that well up. Tears are a gift from deep inside. "There is a sacredness in tears. They are not the mark of weakness, but of power. They speak more eloquently than ten thousand tongues. They are the messengers of overwhelming grief, of deep contrition, and of unspeakable love," wrote Washington Irving.

Remember and re-experience the good memories, if any, connected to this loss.

Acknowledge the pain and hurt of the bad memories.

Recognize whatever unfinished business is connected to this loss.

Accept the fact that your life does go on despite your loss and grief.

Make peace with the "new normal" that your loved one will always be missing. Florence, a 60-year-old woman in recovery from compulsive overeating, ruefully acknowledged, "I understand that my husband died. Yet I can't accept that he's never coming back! Those feel like two different realities."

Decide to get help if depression/anxiety/self blame/or any addictions are ruling your life.

Integrate a ritual or create a memorial, to honor your loss.

When her beloved German shepherd died, Norah had an artist draw a three-dimensional figure of Lucky that "greets" you at her front door.

My own little ritual of paying tribute to my mother occurs each time I land at a New York airport following a trip. My mother would always be sitting by her phone anxiously awaiting our arrival. I would always call her from the airport and announce, "Hi, Mama, we're home!" I knew she waited by the phone eager for reassurance that we hadn't been hijacked, hadn't contracted leprosy, or weren't lying at the bottom of the ocean. Waves of sadness always descend on me in the airport now that there is no mother to call. So, my husband and I say out loud to the universe as we march off to get our luggage, "Hi, Mama, we're home!"

Cultivate other secure relationships, such as a support group or thera-py, which will encourage you to take good care of yourself without the crutch of emotional eating.

As we recover from grief, we find inner signposts that may illus-trate our progress. Glenn, a widower and in recovery from compulsive overeating, tells his story:

"My wife, Camille, and I always loved to go out to eat. We would go to this local restaurant in our neighborhood, Aubergine. That's French for eggplant. After Camille died, for a year and a half, I had this series of dreams of the two of us going to Aubergine for dinner. It was sooth-ing and comforting as if she were still with me, at least in my dreams.

"Then two years after her death, my dream changed: We went back to Aubergine, but they had changed the name. The restaurant's new name was Au Revoir. That is French for goodbye. Then I realized that Au Revoir also means 'til we meet again.' The dream felt like my wife was telling me to move on with my life, that we would see each other again, but now was the time for me to begin a new life without her. The dream made me sad, but I also found it amusing—Camille was sending me a message from heaven!"

As Judith Viorst writes, "So perhaps the only choice we have is to choose what to do with our dead: To die when they die. To live crippled. Or to forge, out of pain and memory, new adaptations. Through mourning we acknowledge that pain, feel that pain, live past it. Through mourning we let the dead go and take them in. Through mourning we come to accept the difficult changes that loss must bring—and then we begin to come to the end of mourning."[7]

Grieving the Loss of an Eating Disorder

As emotional eaters begin to recover, they need to grieve the loss of their best friend and enemy (their "frenemy") of bingeing, purging, starving, and chronic dieting. People often experience grief when they recover from their eating problems because they lose a tried and true way of soothing themselves, a way of giving meaning and focus to their life, a well-worn way of coping with stress, and the magical belief that weight loss will solve all their problems, repair their self-esteem, and help them feel happier. Grief includes the realization of how much wasted time, energy, money, and obsessing the eating disorder has consumed.

Eventually, through the process of healing, we need to part from our eating problems, honor the help they have provided, wave good-bye, and go our separate ways.

This farewell does engender grief as the question remains: "Who am I without my eating disorder?"

Rose Ann has struggled with binge eating disorder, anorexia, and laxative abuse. In her poem, written as she emerges from the bondage of her eating disorders, she portrays the transition from an eating disordered identity to recovering the vitality of living. She captures the confusion, the hope, the vision of how life could be, as well as an acknowledgement of what it has been like living under the tyranny of an eating disorder.

> *Who Am I Without My Eating Disorder?*
> Rose Ann F.
>
> *Who am I without my eating disorder?*
> *I am the dirt on which you walk,*
> *Or am I the ground for which things grow?*
>
> *Who am I without my eating disorder?*
> *I am the rose about to wilt,*
> *Or am I the bud who needs to bloom?*
>
> *Who am I without my eating disorder?*
> *I am the sky that brings such darkness,*
> *Or am I the dawn that brings the light?*
>
> *Who am I without my eating disorder?*
> *I am damaging thunder that brings the storm,*
> *Or am I the rain that brings the rainbow?*
>
> *Who am I without my eating disorder?*
> *I am the fire burning destructively hot,*
> *Or am I the flame that wants to glow?*
>
> *Who am I without my eating disorder?*
> *I am the mouth that craves to eat,*
> *Or am I the lips seeking a kiss so sweet?*

Who am I without my eating disorder?
I am the tears that carry sorrow,
Or am I the tears that set you free?

Who am I without my eating disorder?
I am the eyes that refuse to see,
Or am I searching just for me?

Who am I without my eating disorder?
I am the heart that anxiously skips a beat,
Or am I the pulsing rhythm in my feet?

Who am I without my eating disorder?
I am the life that waits for death,
Or am I the child still unborn
Who waits first breath
To greet new dawn?

The more you run away from intense emotions, the more your eating problems run after you. Grief must be witnessed to be healed. Therapy can help to unfreeze grief. You learn that your pain is not the whole of who you are. Tears thaw grief. Shared pain is soothed pain.

Food for Thought
To chronicle your own history of loss and grief, create a time line from birth to now. Include any rupture, disruption, change, loss, family death or turmoil, significant illness, accident, or violence that occurred to you.

Then, chronicle your time line history with weight and eating disorders.

1. Are there any parallels between these two time lines? Can you relate an upsurge of eating problems to the times of loss or grief?

Doreen made an abridged time line and described it to me: "I actually made a graph of all the losses and changes in my life, then I superimposed my eating disorder history on top of it. Here is what I learned:

- When I was five years old, I was a normal weight kid. Then my parents moved into a house of our own in the suburbs. The photos after that move showed me getting heavier and heavier. I imagine I felt bereft to leave my little friends behind; they were the very first friends I ever had. My mother may have been more socially isolated in the new house because she didn't drive, and my father had more financial responsibilities with the mortgage. I think the heightened anxiety level in my house began fueling my compulsive overeating.

- I had an abortion when I was 24. My guilt, confusion, and shame led to another upsurge of compulsive bingeing in which I gained 30 pounds.

- When I was 40, my older brother was diagnosed with leukemia. As he became more emaciated, I went through a period of anorexia. Part of me really enjoyed the self-control of starvation. Brad died two years later, and my anorexia continued until I went into treatment. Treatment helped me to eventually start eating again, even though a part of me really prefers being anorexic to being normal. Just a part of me, though."

2. If I open my heart to pain, what is my biggest fear?

3. What do I lose if I keep it locked up?

4. How does my emotional eating help keep my pain under wraps?

5. And, as Rose Ann's poem asks, "Who am I without my eating disorder?"

1 Judith Viorst, *Necessary Losses* (Simon & Schuster, 1984), 15.

2 Elizabeth Kübler-Ross, a pioneer in the study of grief and mourning, describes in her book *On Grief and Grieving* how she became involved in this field. As a little girl, her family raised rabbits for food on their farm. Elizabeth had a favorite rabbit, Blackie, who her father eventually insisted be taken to the butcher for slaughter. Elizabeth, aged seven, was the one to take Blackie. After the butcher slaughtered the bunny, he told Elizabeth, "Too bad you didn't wait a couple of days. Blackie was pregnant and about ready to have babies." Elizabeth brought the dead rabbit home, its body still warm in the bag, and watched as her family ate the rabbit for dinner that night. Her heart was broken. "That night at dinner when my family ate Blackie, in my eyes they were cannibals. But I would not cry for this bunny or anyone else for almost forty years." Dr. Kübler-Ross later considered this event pivotal in her future interest in grief and mourning. Elizabeth Kübler-Ross and David Kessler, *On Grief and Grieving* (Scribner, 2005), 212.

This story is of particular interest to me, since I have heard many traumatic stories from eating disorder patients over the years about their intense grieving for the pets they deeply loved:

"Our cat had kittens and my mother flushed them down the toilet."

"My stepfather furiously kicked my dog Molasses until she bled. She died."

"My parakeet flew away when I was a little girl, and no one helped me look for him. I searched the neighborhood all by myself. I was so lonely."

In *French Toast for Breakfast* I recounted a story from a patient named Jenny that reveals the deep connection we can feel with animals:

Jenny's father had died from a drug overdose when she was five. "When I was ten," she said, "I had an experience that was unbearable to me. My mother had just come out of a drug rehabilitation program. She and I found a baby robin on the sidewalk with a broken wing and we brought it inside to nurse it back to health. My mother put the bird on the stove and turned the heat on low to warm him up, but when I came home from school, the bird was lying dead on the stove. She had forgotten to turn the heat off. I felt destroyed, and no one could understand the depth of my reaction. People said 'But, Jenny, it was just a bird.'

"When I came to the eating support group 30 years later and began telling my story and my struggles with overeating, those memories of the bird came back. It occurred to me that I had felt like this little bird—that despite all my mother's good intentions, she was unable to really care for anyone, herself included. These memories of the bird made me experience for the first time the shock and fear I had felt about my father's death. The little robin had seemed so tender and helpless. That bird was like my tender self that had to go underground with food because I could not trust anyone to take good care of me." Mary Anne Cohen, *French Toast for Breakfast* (Gürze Books, 1995), 170.

3 Hope Edelman, *Motherless Daughters.* (Da Capo Press, 2006), 19.

4 Thornton Wilder, *The Bridge of San Luis Rey,*1927.

5 Glenn Schiraldi, Ph.D., *Post-Traumatic Stress Disorder Sourcebook* (McGraw Hill, 2009), 193.

6 Hope Edelman, *Motherless Daughters.*

7 Judith Viorst, *Necessary Losses, 264.*

3. The Inner World of the Emotional Eater

Introduction: The Inner World of the Emotional Eater   54
Anorexia Nervosa   56
Bulimia Nervosa   71
Exercise Bulimia   89
Binge Eating Disorder   96
Obesity   112
Night Eating Syndrome   134
Men and Eating Disorders   142
Pregnancy and Eating Disorders   147
Older Women, Body Image, and Eating Disorders   152

Introduction: The Inner World of the Emotional Eater

The inner world of the emotional eater reduces all conflicts and problems of life into one single obsession: "I'm fat. I'm ugly. I need to lose weight."

Life for all of us is at times confusing, exuberant, contradictory, hopeful, messy, joyful, hurtful, and disappointing. Sometimes it's hard to be a human! We all search for ways to manage life on a daily basis. For the anorexic, bulimic, and compulsive overeater, the ultimate coping mechanism for all of life's uncertainties and frustrations revolves around eating and weight loss.

Emotional eaters simplify their inner confusing feelings by focusing on fat/thin, good/bad, black/white, either/or. Life then becomes structured, organized, and with purpose. Emotional eaters shift their pain from their heart to their stomach, and crystallize inner emotional anguish into feeling fat.

The Story of Brenda

Brenda was a beautiful, exotic looking woman in her late 30s, with long black hair and a slender body.

"Tell me what brings you here," I asked, "and how I can help."

"Two months ago," she began, "I had a double mastectomy. At that time my husband, Mark, left me for another woman. I realized he must have been seeing her for a while. My daughter, Sonia, the one who helped me through all this, is leaving next month for college in California. Now I have no one."

"And your family?" I asked.

"Both my parents are dead. They died in a car crash when I was 12. Then I went to live with my grandmother. She died when I was 17, and that's when I married Mark. Now I have no one."

She stared straight ahead, lost in reverie. The image of her parents' violent death, her mastectomies, and all her other losses was overwhelming.

"Brenda," I said, "you've been through so much. How would you like me to help you?"

She straightened up suddenly and said with determination, "I'm here because I'm fat and I need to lose weight!"

The language of pain comes in many dialects. Emotional eating problems and the fear of being fat is one such dialect in which we recruit our bodies to express what we cannot utter in words. Our eating problems become a vehicle to communicate matters of the heart that have no other channel. The language of food and fat is a symbolic one, a way to express our inner emotional battles over feelings of emptiness and fullness, vulnerability and protection, urge and restraint, desire and despair.

When we cannot express the depth of pain we carry inside, we transform our emotional suffering into physical suffering. This obsession with food and fat is often a shorthand way of expressing much deeper layers of yearning and anguish.

Brenda had been assaulted by so many massive losses in her life that she could not bear to face her grief, rage, and abandonment. Her wish to lose weight was a safe, clear way to express her pain—a language so many people speak.[1]

Emotional eaters struggling with anorexia, bulimia, or binge eating believe that trusting food is safer than trusting people, loving food is safer than loving people. Food never leaves you, never rejects you, never laughs at you, never abuses you, never dies. Food is the only relationship where *we* get to say when, where, and how much. No other relationship complies with our needs so absolutely.

As Marlene Boskind-White and William White write, the eating disordered person is "locked in the past, paralyzed in the present, and fearful of the future."[2] The healing work is to unlock the past, revitalize the present and create hope for the future.

The therapy of the emotional eater is to enable her to feel whole inside herself, with a more expansive, richer experience of life. During her recovery, Brenda hung a picture on her refrigerator—a rainbow ranging from black to white with varying hues of gray. It was to remind her of her more nuanced self-image rather than "my food and body is my only problem in life."

Anorexia Nervosa

"If only we could get my daughter (son, wife) to eat, we could beat this anorexia."

"The cure for my daughter's anorexia is so simple. I tell her, 'Just pick up the damn fork and eat!'"

"Can't he see what an ugly scarecrow he's become?"

Anorexia is about food and not about food. An anorexic person may restrict and avoid food to the point of starvation and even death. (This disease has the highest mortality rate of any psychiatric illness).[3] But, essentially, anorexia is not about food. It is about a person's attempt to solve emotional problems through self-starvation. This curious interplay that anorexia (and all eating disorders) is about food and also not about food is what makes the recovery from these disorders so challenging.

Our society glamorizes anorexia nervosa. We look admiringly at the photos of starving, waif-like models on magazine covers. We envy the so-called "X-ray" women of high society. We get jealous of the woman working out on the treadmill next to us at the gym in the size 2 shorts.

What is anorexia? Who gets it? And why do we envy someone who is good at starving herself?

Anorexia nervosa comes from the Greek word *orexy* meaning "hunger" and the prefix *an* meaning "lack of." *Nervosa* refers to the fact that this illness is emotional (nervous) in origin. Although anorexia literally means "lack of hunger," anorexics *are*, in fact, hungry. Their illness is about the *denial* of their hunger.[4]

Anorexics wage a battle against hunger, eating, and their body size by vigilantly restricting calories, practicing grueling exercise regimes, and often maintaining strange food rituals, such as only eating white foods or chewing gum incessantly. Occasionally, when hunger reasserts itself, the anorexic will binge on the foods she denies herself and then may make herself throw up. Her remorse and self-loathing following a binge leads to her increased rigidity over her food intake. Then the vicious cycle of starving, followed by possible bingeing and purging, begins again.

Despite the stereotypical picture, not all anorexics are female, or young, poorly functioning, or physically ill. An anorexic may be a successful student, married, a parent, have a good job, or even, as in the case of one of my patients, a physician. Despite these possible accomplishments in the outside world, she (or he) is beset with anxiety about eating, fat, calories, exercise, weight, and food and willfully restricts her intake. These preoccupations are just the tip of the iceberg, masking core inner problems of faulty self-esteem and identity. (The anorexic's willful self-starvation and fear of fat defines the eating disorder, as opposed to someone who may temporarily lose interest in eating and lose weight during a period of depression.)

Anorexia generally emerges in the early teen years, but the seeds of this disorder are planted in childhood. The child who later becomes anorexic hates her inner neediness and her dependency on her family. To counter this neediness, she starves herself which is her way of proclaiming, "Look how strong I am. I have no needs. I don't need food. I don't need nourishment. I don't need anyone. I have triumphed over my weaknesses and now I am in control." In her mind, to be fat and overweight is an admission to the world about her shameful, ugly secret—that she is a greedy and hungry little girl.

An eating disorder is a "needing disorder" that has been diverted through food. Underneath the fear of fat and the fear of eating lies the bigger anxiety of giving in to *emotional* hunger: needing attention, needing care, needing to be cuddled, needing to be listened to, to be tucked in at night, to have her hair brushed. Starving equals self-control and strength, and so starving becomes the pseudo-solution to resolve emotional fears. The anorexic "binges" on deprivation.

Hilde Bruch, a psychiatrist and pioneer in the treatment of eating disorders in the 1970s, describes how in the case of the anorexic "the eating function is misused in an effort to solve or camouflage problems of living. For the eating disorder patient, weight loss is thought of as 'medicine' for all that ails her. . . . Anorexics "suffer from severe dissatisfaction about themselves and their lives, and they transfer this dissatisfaction to the body. The body is then treated like something foreign that needs to be protected against getting 'fat.'" And this leads to the "relentless pursuit of thinness."[5]

The Themes of Anorexia

More than any other eating disorder patient, anorexics resist treatment. They want to be left alone to lose even more weight. Helping anorexics recover can be a complicated struggle. Such was the case of Emma.

Emma: Resistant to Help

Before I ever met her, Emma had seven past hospitalizations in her teens for anorexia. I am outside my house when Emma, age 22, comes for her appointment. We have already been working together for some time at this point. As we walk up the outside stone steps of my brownstone office, Emma's heel catches on the top step and she falls down the whole flight with tremendous force. Her knee is scraped and bleeding, she looks dazed. I call out, "Oh, my gosh, Emma, are you all right?" Without a whimper or crying out, Emma picks herself up, acting as if nothing has happened. As I observe her tight-lipped stoicism, I learn so much about the ingredients that have formed Emma's anorexia.

Emma is the oldest of 12 children. Her mother, overwhelmed by so many children, and her father, desperately working to support his family, have unwittingly communicated to their daughter that her needs are an unwanted burden. Early on, she became "mother's little helper" to the other children and often nursed her mother through various medical crises.

Emma prides herself on how little she required growing up; her goal was to spare her mother any extra work. Emma's professed lack of needing any help has allowed her to feel powerful, independent, grown-up, and self-sufficient. Early on, she received praise for her maturity, even though that "maturity" was rooted in silencing and re-pressing her emotional hunger and not from true emotional develop-ment. Emma's refusal to eat, her striving to have no needs (and no fat), became her badge of worth. Anorexic emaciation proved to herself and the world that she could practically live on air, without requiring any nurturing or nourishment from her family or others. She is con-sumed by an ongoing attempt to starve out her inner badness—her secret voracious needs.

While most teenagers enjoy trying out new independence, de-fining their unique identity, exploring their sexuality with curiosity, the anorexic flounders and retreats to a world of isolation and obses-sion about weight and calories. Fearful of growing up, the anorexic "grows down," stalled midway between childhood and adulthood. She is stuck at the crossroads of life. The anorexic girl is Sleeping Beauty, her emerging self lying dormant, hidden under a psychological cocoon of brambles, dreading the kiss of the Prince whom she fears will awak-en her.

When the pre-anorexic girl (or boy) hits puberty, she realizes time is marching on, she is growing up, and there is no turning back. The hope that one day it will be *my* turn to be taken care of grows fainter, as she is now expected to assume more adult responsibilities. Her pre-mature maturity, her self-reliant armor starts to crack, and she retreats to anorexia as an attempt to freeze time. Ironically, by starving herself, she regresses to that very dependent child who now seriously needs the care of others she tried so hard to do without. Her fragile body comes to mirror her fragile inner sense of self. Anorexia is reminiscent of the Spanish song, "Clock, please stop ticking off the hours. Make this moment last forever."

Emma is one of the most difficult patients I have ever worked with. With seven hospitalizations for anorexia and bulimia from age 14 on, her life could best be described as "Girl Interrupted." Emma came to see me at age 19, already married with a baby, because she secretly continued starving and vomiting.

Emma's posture with me was sullen, hostile, and uncommunicative. Nothing I said was helpful. Nothing I did was helpful. Nothing I didn't say was helpful. Nothing I didn't do was helpful. And at the end of every session, Emma would loudly slam my front door with a resounding bang.

When I questioned her about that, she corrected me by saying, "I don't slam your door. I just let it slam behind me. There's a big difference."

I found her answer clever, amusing, and annoying. But I was also aware that the door-slam was the equivalent of her vomiting me out forcefully at the end of each session. Her behavior was saying, "I don't want to be here. You are not important. When you dismiss me at the end of the session, I'll show you how little I care about that. Good bye and good riddance." And yet we persevered. She kept coming religiously to her sessions. And I kept showing up to attentively listen, be curious, and learn about her.

Working with Emma made me feel discouraged and unhelpful. And because I had often experienced these same feelings in my relationship with my mother, Emma also made me angry! Perhaps knowing that all her previous therapy and hospitalizations had not really healed her made me less anxious about having to be the one to finally rescue her. I came to recognize my sense of inadequacy with Emma was really a reflection of how she felt in her own life—ineffective, inadequate, and unimportant. By her refusal to take me in, she was inducing me to experience her inner world.

I decided to tolerate my "inadequacy" and just observe her efforts to devalue me. I studied how and when she undermined me as a way to understand her internal workings.[6]

In one session, we were speaking about old age. "When you're an old lady, I'll take you in to live with me and take good care of you," Emma says. I was astonished by her "offer," since she never had shown me any warmth or demonstrated that I was important to her in any way. I understood her offer to "take me in" as meaning that *emotionally* she was beginning to take me in.

And I recognized in the role-reversal script she created that she was the mother and nurturer, while I was the helpless, little old lady needing her care. This was a mirror image of how she experienced her own childhood with her mother—a role reversal where she cared for her mother and not the other way around.

I asked how she would take care of me. And I teased her about whether she would feed me as little food as she fed herself. We began laughing and kidding each other. Some ice was broken, and we began having a new way of relating—through laughter. This freed us up.

At times, when Emma particularly irritated me, I began to dramatically raise my eyes to heaven and proclaim, "You are so impossible!" I now felt comfortable venting my aggravation directly to her in *words* in the hope she would join me and use *words* to express herself and her hostilities. But her chronic self-expression through starving and vomiting and door-slamming continued on and on.

Then, because of some new-found openness, Emma began relating experiences from her childhood, filled with deprivation and sadness. Rather than just sticking to the "bare bones" of what she told me, Emma was now beginning to "flesh out" her story. Because she was the oldest child, Emma often had to care for her 11 siblings alongside her mother. Her mother never sang her a lullaby nor read her a bedtime story. Her reaction, "I can do without," made her less vulnerable and less disappointed.

When Emma was nine, she deeply yearned for a Cabbage Patch baby doll. A little doll of her own. So unusual that she wanted anything for herself.

Her aunt agreed to buy the doll. Finally, she would have a doll of her own, but it was not freely given. Her aunt requested that Emma pay her back. Emma, in effect, had to buy the doll for herself. And so, once again, she had to act like a grownup.

She told me this story with no emotion, but tears jumped to my eyes. I felt the sorrow for her that she could not feel for herself. It was too dangerous for Emma to own that sorrow and deprivation. There were too many episodes and they reached too close to the bone. Her self-starvation numbed and blocked out dangerous feelings, memories, hurts, needs, desires, yearnings, anger. When you reduce your whole emotional world to "I'm fat and need to lose weight," there is little room for any other feelings.

Emma's story provoked in me the sadness she had never permitted herself to have, and I fantasized buying her a Cabbage Patch doll. I took note that in my fantasy, I was no longer the helpless old lady nor was she the mother caring for me. I was feeling like the mother who wishes to buy a doll for her little girl. She was letting me take care of her in my fantasy life. The tide was shifting.

She wrote me a letter, "I would love to share some meaningful feelings, thoughts with you. There is a particular pain in being unable to put them into words. Just try to understand me in a way deeper than words, beyond words. So I'll communicate in silence. Other than the two most important words, 'Thank you.'"

Yet she continued to starve and throw up and slam my door loudly.

Our unconscious nonverbal, communication continued in surprising ways. She was seeing me twice a week and, in a burst of tenderness to her, I thought silently to myself in our session, "I wish Emma could come to therapy three times a week." Simultaneously she says out loud to me: "I hate therapy!" At the very moment I was wanting another "portion," she was spitting and starving it out!

Me: "And here I was thinking, I wanted to see you three times a week."

Emma: "Well, that's basically the same thing as me hating therapy."

We laughed heartily at the absurdity of our different positions. Me, the therapist, who enjoys eating, did not have any problem wanting another serving. Emma, the anorexic client, frightened of hunger— physical or emotional—was all prepared to starve me out. Yet, we recognized that we were feeling mutually tender to each other in our own ways.

Emma writes me a poem, spelling out the word "therapist:":

> *This is easier written than said*
> *How to express some thoughts in my head.*
> *Every now and then you deserve to know*
> *Really how I appreciate you so.*
> *Actually I do like coming here*
> *Promising myself I'll try to share*
> *I know I could be quite a pain*
> *Surprised you haven't gone insane*
> *Totally Terrific Therapist!*

After much mutual spilling of blood, sweat, tears, and her vomit, Emma allowed herself to slowly develop a caring attachment to me. She has been free from starving and vomiting for a number of years. She has had two more children. She feels more secure with her husband than ever before. She returned to school for the first time since the onset of her hospitalizations for bulimia at age 14 and has graduated from college.

Girl Interrupted has become Girl Flourishing.

No more starving or vomiting.

She still continues to slam the door.

Ginny: I Am Fat = I Have Needs = I Am Bad

Ginny is an 18-year-old, 82-pound anorexic patient. Like Emma, she describes her lifelong shame about requiring any care from her parents. Ginny makes this startling revelation, "When I think about being a baby and being dependent on my mother even to change my diaper, it fills me with revulsion. I wish I were born knowing how to change my own diaper so as not to feel so disgusting and weak."

Ginny's parents were both alcoholics. As a consequence, Ginny developed a fear of dependency and neediness because she had never felt safe and secure about her normal and natural childhood needs.

A child's insecurity may develop in any family that is consumed and distracted by problems. The issue could be illness, or a death, addiction, financial problems, depression, or sexual abuse, or because other children in the family have their own competing demands. In these various situations, parents become overwhelmed and cannot adequately nurture their child. The child becomes emotionally hungry. Faced with the ongoing prospect of feeling deprived, she begins to suppress her needs for nurturance. She trains herself to want less and less. In resisting food, she gains a sense of control over her life. Food and fat are the enemy; her self-starving becomes her identity—a badge of virtue, strength, and triumph.

The anorexic appears victorious. But it is a hollow victory as her life becomes more constricted. She is consumed by the need to lose more weight and achieve self-sufficiency, and loses sight of living a full, enjoyable life with health and verve.

Helping Ginny return to normal eating was achieved by a team of therapists who became like a second-chance family to her. This included treatment by a psychotherapist, a physician, a psychiatrist who prescribed medication, a nutritionist, and hospitalization. Sometimes it takes a village to heal an anorexic!

Each patient requires her own personal treatment plan which may also include family therapy. Because anorexia can be a life-threatening disease, careful professional monitoring of food and weight often needs to continue for a lengthy period of time to prevent the anorexic from slipping back to her familiar patterns of refusing to eat.[7]

Gaining weight does not mean the anorexic is cured. Of course, weight gain is critical because malnutrition affects not only health but psychological functioning. But restoring weight is only half the battle. Unless the person embarks on a journey to connect with her inner world of feelings, the underlying problems causing anorexia will continue to fuel the eating disorder. Ongoing psychotherapy helps the anorexic become self-reflective and curious about her fear of fat and more self-compassionate and accepting of her world of emotions and human imperfections.

Ginny's recovery included helping her make peace with her deep need for others and how this had led to a distorted desire to control her appetite. Fearful of losing their daughter, Ginny's parents were motivated to enter treatment and work on their own struggles with alcohol and marital fidelity.

Harriet: The Need for Ownership

Harriet is an anorexic girl in her 20s weighing 90 pounds. During our second session together, the air conditioner is running and Harriet puts on her sweater and buttons it up. "Are you cold?" I ask. "I don't know," she answers.

It is astonishing that she does not know. From childhood, the anorexic often fails to develop full awareness or trust in her feelings and beliefs. She may lose touch with her body sensations—hunger, fullness, fatigue, sexuality. This, in turn, leads to self-doubt and problems with self-esteem and identity. Her need for some kind of power over her internal confusion leads her to starve her body. And so it was with Harriet.

As Harriet's therapy progressed she began to describe how her relationship with her father often caused her bewilderment. "Dad wanted me to become a doctor," she said. "He shoved this idea down my throat constantly. It got to the point I wasn't sure if I wanted that for myself or whether I just wanted to please him. He was an authoritarian person who would declare things like, 'It's lunch time. I know you must be hungry.' But I was never sure if I really was hungry."

Then, one day after many sessions of therapy together, Harriet reported to me the following: "Dad and I were sitting at home just recently, and I said I was cold and could he turn up the heat? He responded, 'No. You are not cold.'

"I was startled. A light bulb went off inside me, and I got angry. I realized most normal parents would say, 'Well, *I'm* not cold' or 'Are you *really* cold?' But Dad announced that he knew I was not cold as if he could read me better than I could read myself. At that point I determined never to allow anyone other than myself to evaluate whether I was cold or hot or hungry or full or sleepy or wanting to be a doctor. I vowed to learn to tune in to what *I* think and what *I* feel. I don't want anyone else's opinions to overpower me or intrude on my experiences; I need to figure out where Dad ends and *I* begin. I need to take ownership over my own body. 'Ownership' has become my new favorite word!"

Harriet's anorexia is a clear example of how anorexia is about food—her need to control through self-starvation—and also not about food. Through the therapy journey of discovering her inner self and bringing her confusion and feelings into the clear light of day, Harriet gradually became more self-assertive and improved her relationship to food, eating, and her own special self.

Grace: Inner Confusion

Grace, another anorexic girl in her late teens, reveals her confusion in a different way. During one of our sessions she describes the sympathetic way she handled a problem that her cousin had confided in her. I say to her, "You were very compassionate to your cousin. You felt empathy for your cousin's troubles, but you find it so hard to show the same compassion for yourself."

"But, is it a good thing or a bad thing to be compassionate?" Grace asks.

It is astonishing she does not know. Grace is confused about whether compassion is good or bad and is uncertain if hunger is good or bad, eating is good or bad, her needs are good or bad, sexuality is good or bad. Like Emma and Harriet, Grace shows an uncertainty and lack of trust in herself.

Grace came from a family that was overwhelmed by caring for her deaf brother Timmy. Little time or energy was available to focus on "hearing" Grace—her needs, her feelings, her wishes. And so, once again like Emma and Harriet, she determined that by minimizing her eating she could prove to herself that she was strong, independent, and without needs. She reduces all her feelings to "I am fat," which is shorthand for "I don't know or trust myself."

Our work together focuses on helping Grace listen to her inner self. Then one day she tells me, "I was swimming laps in a pool and decided to cut the workout short. I was tired, and I had enough swimming for the day." This is the first time since we began working together that Grace identifies a sensation in her body. And she listens to it. And she responds.

This may seem like an insignificant detail to most people, but for Grace this is significant progress. Up to that point, she was deaf to her body's signals of fatigue, hunger, or fullness. In time, Grace developed a partnership with her body, the partnership of listening to herself the way she never had with her family. As she "heard" her hunger more clearly, she wanted to respond and feed herself.

Grace's anorexia was about food—her self-starvation—and also not about food. Only by taking the journey inward and listening to her needs was she able to heal and begin to feed and nourish herself.

Grace's recovery touches on the three steps of self-care that anorexics and all eating disorder patients need to learn:

1. Identifying their inner feelings.
2. Listening to them.
3. Responding to them.

Additional Themes in Recovery from Anorexia

> *This plant would like to grow*
> *And yet be embryo;*
> *Increase, and yet escape*
> *The doom of taking shape . . .*
> —Richard Wilbur, "Seed Leaves"

A Recovery Crisis

As the person with anorexia begins to enjoy and want the connection with the healing therapist—maybe one of the first times she has felt listened to—she will often go through a crisis. She says to herself, "If I'm not anorexic and starving myself any longer, I have no good reason to be in therapy." And so the anorexic may cling to her illness because she does not want to lose the caring relationship with the therapist. She may not feel entitled to receive help unless she is suffering from an eating disorder which then makes her feel justified to continue treatment.

I often say to my patients, "I'd really like to get to know you without anorexia. Maybe there are other important things we can talk about beside food and eating."

Emma asks, "Even though I'm not starving anymore, I like coming here. Does that mean I'm not healthy? Wouldn't a healthy person want to stop therapy?"

Clearly she is looking for permission to continue but still feels bad about what she considers her neediness. I respond, "A healthy person does what she wants—as long as it does not hurt herself or anyone else. A healthy person focuses on what she wants rather than worrying about how she assumes the world may judge her."

Another fear of the recovering anorexic: In her mind, to get better means she now must grow up 100 percent and become completely self-reliant. "The prospect of doing well or gaining weight is dreaded because growing up means loss, loneliness, and helplessness. Growing up means giving up the fantasy of being able to return to early childhood and this time having it come out right. In her fantasy, the anorexic can 'go home,' start over, and this time around be a perfect child to perfect parents. To give up this fantasy is to reconcile herself to the fact that there is no going back and starting over; this fills her with depression. The therapist must help her tolerate this depression."[8]

Relinquishing anorexia can feel like a loss. Getting better may instill some fear about how to handle feelings in the future without the crutch of self-starvation. Recognizing and anticipating and talking about these worries is an important stage of recovery.

Self Empathy

Another rarely discussed factor that fosters recovery involves the capacity to feel sorry for one's self. Common "wisdom" instructs us not to feel sorry for ourselves because it is too self-indulgent. But I believe sorrow for oneself marks a turning point in recovery. If the anorexic can feel compassion for the little girl inside her who was deprived and hurt, she becomes kinder and more willing to take care of herself. Most people grieve for what they have lost; the anorexic needs to grieve for what she never had—comfort and empathy in her early family life.

Emma needs to experience her childhood pain without running away. Instead of numbing her hurt by starvation, she needs to grieve the carefree childhood she never had. Ginny needs to grieve for the alcoholism of her parents and their impaired ability to take care of her. Harriet needs to grieve for the self that was hijacked by her father's domination. Grace needs to grieve for her childhood that was inadvertently lost to Timmy's deafness.

As Hilde Bruch described, anorexia is not just an illness of weight and dieting but an "illness of inner self-awareness, of inner emptiness, inner loneliness, and inner unworthiness."[9]

As the therapist helps the anorexic "flesh out" her life story, the person hopefully comes to accept her hunger for human connection and her hunger for food. She experiences the birth of her genuine self, a self that can provide her with companionship, verve, vitality, identity, and comfort in her life. She learns to trust and enjoy her opinions, feelings, and beliefs.

Bulimia Nervosa: Self Harm from the Inside Out
The worst loneliness is not to be comfortable with yourself.
—Mark Twain

Megan: Bulimic with Food/Bulimic with Relationships
"You are my eighth therapist," Megan, a pretty 24-year-old woman, announces cheerfully as she enters my office. "Not one of them ever helped me."

I am surprised at the triumphant note in her voice. Why would this girl feel triumph at defeating all eight therapists who tried to help her? I think to myself, "And I'm sure I won't be your last therapist either. And I bet you're bulimic—who else would consume and spit out so many therapists by the age of 24?" I am surprised at my quick and uncharacteristic coolness toward Megan.

"I have been bulimic since I was 15," Megan states, "but my bulimia is worse because I'm in an emotional crisis. My father recently died. That's no big deal—I was never close to him. And he left me five million dollars."

"Some crisis!" I think to myself.

"But," Megan continues, "he left my two older brothers ten million dollars each."

I'm stunned. I'm speechless. Even my inner voice has no comment.

"My Dad decided to leave them more, I guess, because they're married with children and I'm single. I guess he thought they deserved the money more than me. So, on one hand, I am grateful. After all, nobody I know ever inherited five million. But I'm also furious. I feel rejected. Am I selfish to want more? Am I justified? Am I wrong? Am I right? Yes? No? Should I just enjoy what I did get? I really am lucky, after all. But I also feel betrayed. I am pissed off. I can't make up my mind what I should feel. So, I binge, purge, binge, purge, binge, purge. Back and forth. Up and down. Guilty, not guilty. I can't get settled inside myself with all these opposite feelings."

"Well, maybe you don't have to have only one feeling," I suggest. "Why can't you be grateful for inheriting so much money *and* furious that your father divided it unevenly? Why can't you feel lucky *and* gypped at the same time? Can you value what you are getting *and* also be upset that your brothers got more? You are allowed to have *all* these different feelings."

"Really? You mean people can have such totally opposite contradictory feelings? Megan fell silent.

"Welcome to the world of conflict and contradiction," I add. "I'd say you have very good reasons for a lot of different mixed emotions."

As Megan's story unfolds, I also learn that she flits from boyfriend to boyfriend. Her pretty seductiveness enables her to easily get involved in new relationships; she uses her charm as a lure for men's attention and approval. But just as quickly, she becomes disillusioned and invariably pushes them away. She binges and purges on men.

"You are as bulimic with men as you are with food." I point out and add, "And also with therapists." I want to help her see the connection between her binge/purge eating disorder and her binge/purge disorder in relationships. Her bulimia is not just about weight preoccupation, but also a coping method to deal with anxious feelings about getting close to people.

Although the current worsening of her bulimia was provoked by her anger/guilt/confusion over her inheritance, bingeing and purging has been Megan's way of managing her feelings and food for years.

Slowly she begins to see how her push/pull with food parallels her push/pull in life and relationships. Megan grew up with a mother who became bedridden with the progressive disease lupus; her father was preoccupied with his real estate business and running away from the pain of a disabled wife. Megan's mother abandoned her daughter because of illness; her father because of business preoccupations and emotional avoidance. In a rare sad moment, she describes, "I am always hungry for love, but getting love from my parents was like getting blood from a stone."

Megan turned to her own body for comfort and solace, preoccupied with controlling her food, her weight, her appearance. Rigid diets led to break through bingeing and then vomiting to rid herself of unwanted food and unwanted emotional pain.

As a young teenager, she became sexually active early on, trying to feed her hunger for attention and love. She used her body as a token to trade for affection. In each relationship, as the boy began to know her better, Megan "fired" him before he might "fire" her. Megan's "style" reminds me of the old Italian movie, *Seduced and Abandoned*. She would seduce the man, then abandon him.

This history helped me better understand Megan's engulfing and discarding so many therapists. Before she gets too attached, she "purges" them because of her fear of becoming too connected and needy. She purges them in anticipation of having the rug pulled out from under her, similar to what happened emotionally in her family when her mother got sick. Megan protects herself from the pain of needing by constantly moving on. Therapists, men, girlfriends are ejected before they get to know the real Megan—the emotionally hungry and needy bulimic girl. She is ashamed of the craving little girl living at her core.

Learning about Megan's ambivalence in getting close to people, I now understand my initially cold reaction when she began therapy. I sensed that to protect our beginning relationship from her overly friendly, quick, breezy attachment, I needed to create some equilibrium. I restrained my usual warm, welcoming style and tried to maintain the distance between us. I did not want Megan to feel engulfed or seduced into sharing more with me before she is ready. I try to hold back emotionally and regulate the space between us so Megan does not get too attached too quickly and then need to expel me prematurely. She bonds quickly in an attempt to repair her lonely, damaged self, but then must abandon everybody before the neediness of her inner little girl threatens to overwhelm and destroy the relationship.

We are dancing an emotional cha-cha. When I am moved to reach out emotionally and take a step toward her, I sense her retreat. When she reaches out, I intuitively step back a bit to protect her from getting too close too soon. Together we try to straddle the dilemma between her wish for closeness and her fear of it.

We have found a rhythm of comfortably working together. I want to slowly build her trust as we get to know each other. I want Megan to feel cared about and listened to but in small, tolerable doses, like how you feed a rescued baby kitten with a tiny eyedropper of warm milk. But just as the mistrustful, abandoned kitten may bolt after a few licks of milk, so did Megan bolt after a few months of therapy. Following my two-week vacation, she never came back. No amount of phone calls or e-mails led to her return. I explained into the void of her answering machine how I thought she was running away from her anger/disappointment/abandonment by me, and that we needed to speak about this rather than have her dump me as she had done to so many others. "Please don't purge me out," I entreated.

I was very sorry to see Megan leave in such an abrupt manner. Without a goodbye. I believe she experienced my time away as a painful replay of the frequent physical abandonments by her ill mother and the emotional abandonment of her neglectful father. By leaving me, she evened the score. She was ultimately the one in control of the final leaving.

I hope eventually there will be a therapist #9 and Megan will continue exploring her fear and mistrust of human nurturing and food nourishment. And I hope she will come to believe that there exists consistent caring and love in the world for her to have and to hold and to keep and to trust.

The Who, What, When of Bulimia

In 1914, the first chronicle of a bulimic woman, Ellen West, was published. Her poignant description of her bulimia rings true more than a century later: "My life . . . is filled with dread. Dread of eating, dread of hunger, dread of the dread."[10]

Bulimia nervosa is both a *biological* and *emotional* illness.[11] Some bulimics are fat and some are thin; some binge and purge; some also starve along with bingeing and purging; others purge without bingeing. Some spit out the food before they swallow. Some swallow, bring up the food, and re-swallow repeatedly. Some use laxatives or diuretics. Some cut themselves. Some exercise compulsively. Some take drugs or drink alcoholically. Bulimia encompasses a wide range of behaviors. Some women may binge on buying clothes and then purge by returning them the next day.

Bulimia usually develops as the teenager begins the transition out of adolescence. By focusing on calories, food, weight, and eating, the teenager is able to distract herself from the normal anxieties of growing up, sexual worries, and conflicts around forming an adult identity. The very act of bingeing and purging dulls and anesthetizes difficult internal feelings. The ritual of planning the binge and purge, overeating and vomiting, cleaning up afterward, hiding the evidence, and beginning the cycle again consumes a large amount of time and energy, serving as a detour from the demands of real life. The bulimic's eating cycle starts with ransacking the food: ravage > regret > regurgitate > repent > restrict > repeat.

Depression, alcohol, substance abuse, and anxiety and panic disorders are highly prevalent among bulimics as well as their close family members. This supports the belief that strong family genetic and biochemical causes contribute to all these disorders.

Bulimics tend to be more impulsive than anorexics, more sexually active, often with a history of sexual abuse, and may suffer from post-traumatic stress disorder.

Unlike anorexics, who deny they have a problem, bulimics are aware of being in trouble, but because of shame, guilt, and fear they will often not reach out for help. The thin bulimic sees her slenderness as counterfeit because she has achieved it by "cheating," and so she is terrified to be found out. She feels like a fraud trying to maintain her weight through vomiting.

Bulimia is a form of coping, a creative solution to deal with unmanageable feelings. Vomiting is a violent act that releases tension, purifies the self, blunts the pain. Because the bulimic discharges her feelings through *action,* it is difficult yet crucial to help her *tolerate* and *be* with her emotions, rather than *doing* something about them.

For some people, bingeing and purging does not sufficiently alleviate their inner anguish and anxiety over feelings of emptiness, neediness, abuse, rage, and guilt. When vomiting is not sufficiently cathartic to vent their deep frustrations, bulimics often recruit their bodies in more violent ways to express their anger and destructive emotions. Violence against the self escalates. Pulling one's hair out, picking one's face, burning, skin cutting, compulsively piercing or tattooing, rubbing caustic substances into the skin to prevent wounds from healing, and risky sexual behavior are other forms of using one's body as a "canvas" to act out dark impulses. Since bulimics have not found a satisfying, verbal way to express themselves, they discharge their feelings through their bodies instead.[12] Suicide, obviously, is the ultimate dangerous form of self-harm.

Simone described how when she was a little girl she was prohibited from expressing any resentment to her mother. Instead, when she was frustrated, she would bang her head against the wall. Her mother would lash out and sarcastically demand, "Bang your head harder!" And Simone would obey and do her mother's bidding and bang her head harder. This was the beginning of a lifelong tendency to purge feelings destructively through her body and her bulimia.

Fran: Self-Injury and Bulimia

When I was 18 years old, I studied Spanish at the Universidad de Mexico. On one of my excursions through Mexico City, I visit the Basilica of Guadalupe, devoted to the Virgin of Guadalupe, the patron saint of Mexico. I watch in fascination and horror as hundreds of Mexican faithful crawl slowly and painfully on their knees along a treacherous stone path to pay tribute to the Virgin of Guadalupe. Their knees and palms are lacerated and bleeding. They sacrifice their flesh in this communal religious act of mortification and spiritual cleansing in order to atone for their sins.

A decade later, as an eating disorder therapist, I remember the Basilica of Guadalupe. I think about how we humans often recruit our bodies as the vehicle to express and purge matters of the heart and soul that we cannot utter in words. I recall this experience in my work with Fran.

Fran comes home late from a date and crawls into bed. As she falls asleep, her mother storms into her room and begins kicking her bed, "Where were you? Who were you with? You're a slut!" The mother keeps up this tirade until Fran is crying and cowering under the blankets. Her mother, resentful of any social life that Fran has, attacks her out of jealousy. It is a miracle that Fran has the resilience to have any social life at all. After her mom leaves the room, Fran, in a frenzy of fear, agitation, and rage, takes out her razor knife and cuts her stomach. Slice. Slice. Slice. She has hurt her mother. She is a bad daughter. A selfish and ungrateful daughter.

Fran is bulimic and also compelled to injure herself. When the "remedy" of bingeing and vomiting is not powerful enough to quell her rage and panic, she turns to other stronger methods of hurting herself as punishment for her inner "badness." As we see in Fran's case, she moves from being the victim of her mother's abuse to victimizing herself by self-abuse. Whereas bulimia is self-injury from the inside out, cutting is self-injury from the outside in.

In the television series "Dexter," the title character coins the term "Dark Passenger" to describe his inner invisible devil, the one that drives him to kill people which he must hide from others. Although the average person's Dark Passenger does not involve murder, the bulimic and self-harmer have a buried part of themselves that they want to keep secret, a Dark Passenger of the soul. As June, a bulimic patient stated, "In my recovery, I am moving from my inner demons to daylight."

I have observed that bulimics who injure themselves rarely cry. We are only able to cry when we feel sorrow and empathy for ourselves. These children were taught, "bite the bullet" or "suck it up" or "it is what it is, deal with it" or "you're too sensitive" or "you have to learn to take the good with the bad," "others have it worse," "stop crying or I'll really give you something to cry about." So their tears freeze inside, and their emotions of pain and rage burrow underground. Vomiting and bleeding are all bodily expressions of the numb child who could not cry. As psychotherapist Dr. Sharon Farber writes, "Blood that is deliberately shed may express tears that could not be cried and sorrows that could not be spoken. When the body weeps tears of blood, we need to wonder what terrible sorrows cannot be spoken."[13]

Why does Fran hurt herself with bulimia as well as cutting, a tendency of many eating disordered people? Why would someone who is emotionally anguished and angry want to hurt herself and make the pain even worse?

Fran has no other outlet to discharge and relieve her tension. She has no one to speak with and no words forceful enough to express the depth of her sorrow, loneliness, and rage. Fran punishes herself because she feels guilty for wanting to hurt her mother in revenge. Cutting wipes out her mother's attack on her. "The pain I inflict on myself drowns out what she does to me."

Fran reclaims the power and control away from her mother and declares, "I'm in control of hurting myself. I get to control when, where, and how much."

Physical pain is easier to manage than emotional pain. She can localize the pain on one specific place on her body, rather than feel an amorphous suffering in her soul.

Cutting is "medicine" for her anger, guilt, badness, depression. Cutting, like purging, releases endorphins, the body's natural calming chemicals.

To vent her fury directly at her mother is too dangerous. She loves her mother and does not want her mother to abandon her or punish her even more.

Fran believes, "I am immune to my mother's attack because I can dole it out even worse to myself." She attempts to relieve herself of the original pain caused by her mother through doing something even more painful.

"I cut myself to spite her. She would be worried if she knew the damage I do to myself."

She protects her mother from her aggression.

The pain of cutting "purges" her mind of thoughts of loneliness and abandonment. Fran wants to "cut" her mother out of her life.

When the episode is over, Fran feels release and relief and can go back to sleep, temporarily alleviated from her pain.

I learn all these meanings about Fran's vomiting and cutting because, unlike Megan, she does not bolt from therapy. She calls me her "loony doctor" and takes enough insulting "stabs" at me during the years we work together to satisfy her need to dole out pain. She satisfies some of her need to throw up by "vomiting" on me with her graphic descriptions of the plumbing in her mother's house getting corroded from her puke, by describing the nitty-gritty of her cutting and bleeding rituals, and how she picks her face and squeezes pimples and wounds on her skin.

Whereas many self-injuring bulimics hide their "handiwork," others flaunt their cuts, the bald spots where they have pulled out hair, and the scratching of their face or arms. They demonstrate their inner pain by inflicting these external wounds.

With each self-injuring bulimic, I evaluate whether there is a suicide intention. If a suicide potential exists, the patient needs to be hospitalized and kept safe while she works through the current crisis of destructive self-hatred. Then therapy can resume. With Fran, her cutting is a silent scream that needs to be translated into words.

If Fran announces she has cut herself during the week, I intently ask to see her arms or stomach. Sometimes I touch the cuts on her arm with my finger, sometimes I have cried out in alarm upon seeing them. Then I consult with her about what we are going to do to keep them clean and avoid infection, and we join together like two mothers clucking worriedly over their hurt little girl. I invite her to bond with me to decide what actions to take to heal the cuts. She continues to hurt herself but is allowing me to participate in finding ways to make it better. We are at a transitional bridge—halfway between self-injury and self-preservation, a "bridge over troubled waters."

Dr. Joyce McDougall, whose work focuses on psychosomatic (body/mind) illness, describes: "These psychosomatic processes [of self destructive behavior] derive from inner scripts that were written in early childhood and enacted on 'the theater of the body.'"[14]

I try to involve Fran, as I do all my eating disorder patients, in translating her symptoms from "the theater of the body" into emotional and verbal language. I look at the recent cuts Fran has made on her arm and decide to study them as cryptic hieroglyphics. "What do these scratches say?" I ask her.

"They say, 'Fuck you, Mary Anne Cohen,'" she answers without skipping a beat.

I am delighted! Fran is venting her aggression outward—to me—rather than taking it out on herself. Better a "cutting" comment to me than cutting herself. "Well, I think I see some fine print on your arm that may explain why the scratches say fuck me," I point to some additional redness on her forearm.

Fran looks down on her arm as if she too has gotten on board with wanting to "read" the hieroglyphics. "Oh, yes," she says. "It says that sometimes I wish you were my mother and that makes me feel guilty. You want me to talk about my feelings rather than puking and I like that but I also resent it. My mother doesn't ever try to understand me. It's hard to let you care about me because it makes my mother's meanness feel worse by comparison. See? That's what that scratch says here," she concludes, laughing at her imaginative translation.

Does Fran's bulimia and self-injury magically disappear now? No. But we now have created a new language of communicating. She has taken ownership that her behavior has meaning, which helps her emerge from her lonely isolation and shame. She has put words to her pain. She has allowed me into her private world of pain. Our journey together now continues on more solid footing.[15]

Charlene: Too Much, Too Little, and the Black Jelly Bean
Charlene is a ballet dancer—thin, ethereal, beautiful—who throws up her food multiple times a day. Charlene's father grew up an orphan; her mother, who is anorexic herself, grew up with a distant, alcoholic father. This is a marriage made in emotional heaven—both

husband and wife bond around making do with as little as possible. It has become their lifestyle. Both her parents have experienced scarcity in their growing-up years and deprivation has become their unchallenged comfort zone. Charlene has learned that food and needs are dangerous beyond the bare minimum and that thinness represents an emblem of strength for her family. Whenever she believes she has eaten too much, she must throw it up, give it back as if to prove she didn't really want or need it anyway.

When Charlene shared with her parents her decision to begin therapy, her mother's initial reaction: "I hope they're not going to make you gain too much weight."

Charlene realized her mother's anxiety was misguided. Ballet is one of Charlene's deep, abiding passions and she wants the strength to continue. When someone has a passion beyond the eating disorder, she has a deep reason to latch on to the fight for health and recovery.

When Charlene was a child she loved her ballet teacher, Miss Tara, who became her role model. "We were having a Christmas party at the dance studio with cookies and candy and soda. I saw Miss Tara reach into a bowl of jelly beans and pick out just one jelly bean. It was the only thing she ate that whole evening. She picked the black jelly bean which is the worst-tasting of all. Just one black jelly bean. I admired her discipline and self-control so much. I vowed to be just like her."

"What?" I ask incredulously. "You took as your role model a woman who chose just one black jelly bean? That is so depressing and depriving."

Charlene shakes her head sadly. "I guess Miss Tara was another version of my parents. I thought it was greedy to take plenty of food and nourishment for myself. I learned that message so well from my family, it became engrained."

Charlene, by recognizing her constricted commitment to self-inflicted denial in her life and in her eating, began to rework these inner messages. I believe I became a more enriched role model for her than Miss Tara—more earthy, more lively, more colorful—than her previous narrow world.

Many years have passed since Charlene resolved her bulimia and the struggle to embrace pleasure. Her battle over taking too much versus too little has evolved to discovering what is "just right" for her. I recently received a joyful note from her chronicling how well her life is now going, "I feel like a new person with a deep appreciation of my past, present and future." She adds, "I remember fondly our work together. I remember the fragrance of your breakfast toast when I came for my morning appointments. And I remember loving that blue and white dress of yours with the blue earrings."

I enjoy that Charlene is flourishing and that she has taken in some colorful memories of our time together. She has evolved from that girl who once upon a time admired Miss Tara with her one black jelly bean.

Gloria: Laxatives Were My Lifeline

Gloria writes about her life and shares with me what she has written in her journal: "I have been angry all my life," Gloria begins, "probably from when I was an embryo! My brother, Keith, and I lived in constant fear. Dad was an alcoholic, my mother a rageaholic, and neither seemed happy to be our parents. The violence that went on our house was unbelievable—my father hit my mother and my mother beat me and Keith. Keith and I clung to each other when we were young, but then he found a way out of his pain. Keith came out as gay when he was 13 and by age 20 he was dead from AIDS. I believe Keith allowed himself to get AIDS 'accidentally on purpose.' He knew he was involved in risky behavior, and I really believe he passively committed suicide. He had no other way to deal with how traumatized he felt in his life._

"I realized I also was passively committing suicide. My mother was constantly teasing me and criticizing my weight. I was plump, but not fat. I decided that if I lost weight, maybe she would finally love me more. At 14 I began restrictive dieting, bingeing, and taking laxatives. Laxatives were my lifeline. The evacuation of shit from my body felt so liberating and violent and painful and thrilling. Each time it was like trying to forcefully purge the violence of my family out of my system. Of course, the relief was short-lived, but I would do it over and over again. I loved the power and control and even the pain of expelling waste from my body.

"My college roommate reported my laxative abuse to the school, and they mandated I go to therapy. I was furious to be forced to go, and I lashed out from the minute I arrived at Mary Anne's office. I hated her. I hated therapy and did not want to give up laxatives. I yelled, I screamed, I criticized, and Mary Anne just sat there, self-contained, saying, 'You have a lot of shit inside of you. But those laxatives are not helping you well enough to get all the crap out of your system. So let's talk about what you're doing and what you're feeling.'

"Mary Anne never forced me to stop using them. She did ask me to be monitored by the internist she works with. I felt she understood me by not insisting I go cold turkey as long as I wasn't in medical danger. But I kept fighting with her, with my roommate, with my teachers, and so much anger began spewing out of me. I felt like the devil. Mary Anne challenged me to match the strength of my words and my anger with the force of evacuating with laxatives. I howled with rage and grief and tears. After years of this work, I got so much crap up and out. I began really feeling sorry for myself and what I had been through and also what I had put my body through. In a way, I beat the crap out of myself the same way my mother did. I finally didn't want the laxatives, hardly ever. My anger to Keith for ending his life impelled me to want to rewrite my future and learn how to truly live. I also wanted to be alive to honor his memory.

"How Mary Anne put up with me over all this time, I don't know.

I noticed after several years of working together, Mary Anne had a lot more gray hair than when I began therapy. I asked her whether her gray hair was my fault because I had worn her out by being so impossible. She laughed heartily and answered, 'Could be!' But then she added, 'But I like my gray hair. As you may have noticed, I'm not dying it.' No one had ever laughed *with* me and not at me. She was having fun with me, but not at my expense.

"Something shifted at that point. I shared with Mary Anne my interest in travel and art. She was amazed there were parts of me that hadn't been eaten up alive by all the trauma and laxatives. I felt like we were both beginning to know the whole of me, my genuine self— that there was more to me than just pain and suffering and laxatives. In the past several years, I've made some friends, got a beautiful calico kitten, taken an art class. It can still be rocky at times when my anger gets the best of me, but Mary Anne has pulled me back from the brink and helped me preserve these relationships rather than shitting them out."

To paraphrase Bette Davis, working with Gloria certainly was a bumpy ride. There were times when she provoked me so much that I wanted to evacuate her from my office and my life and flush her down the toilet never to be seen again. Yet she also had her endearing moments, such as when she came to my office singing a laxative advertisement from the 1960s that her mother had sung to her:

If, if, if, nature should forget
Go to your medicine cabinette
Use Ex-Lax, use Ex-Lax
And you'll feel you're living again
You'll feel you're living again.

Her playful nature shone through with her singing, and soon after, in one of the turning points in her recovery, Gloria decided to rescue a kitten from a city shelter. She felt she had some love to give and wanted to nurture a little abandoned creature. She has been a good, attentive mother to Gingerella, her calico cat.

Gloria is one of the most resilient women I have ever met. I admire her tenacity to finally meet life head on without laxatives, bingeing, or other self-abuse.

Laxative Abuse

Laxative abuse, a form of bulimia, is quite dangerous and easy to get hooked on. Many people with binge eating disorder turn to laxatives or enemas in the hope of rushing the food through the intestines to avoid gaining weight. Since most of the calories eaten are absorbed by the small intestine right after eating, using laxatives for weight loss is actually ineffective.

Laxatives are sold over-the-counter and in health stores, giving the impression they are safe. Their names lull a person into believing they are benign: Whole Body Cleanse, Great Regular Organic Tea, Triple Process Total Body Detox and Cleanse, Smooth Move. Who wouldn't want to try to Correct-all that is wrong with their lives?

The danger is that laxative abusers use them in ever-increasing amounts, giving rise to medical complications:

- Constipation.
- Ongoing overstimulation of the intestines from laxative abuse eventually can cause the bowels to become unresponsive.
- Dehydration with possible tremors, weakness, blurry vision, fainting, kidney damage, and, in extreme cases, death.
- Electrolyte imbalance, with possible danger to the heart, nerves, and muscles and risk of death.

Stopping the laxative abuse cycle is best done under the care of a physician for medical management and a psychotherapist for emotional support and psychological insight. After stopping the laxatives, certain measures can aid the transition back to regular elimination:

- Drink six to ten cups of water daily.
- Moderate exercise can stimulate regular bowel movements.
- Regular meals can help the body relearn the normal digestion function. Fruits and vegetables and whole-grain products will help normalize digestion.
- Prepare yourself mentally for feeling bloated, constipation, and *temporary* weight gain as the body readjusts. This does not mean you are getting fat!
- Patience is required. Symptoms of laxative withdrawal can last from three weeks to a month.

Diuretic abuse is another form of purge-related bulimia in which the person with an eating disorder tries to lose weight by using diuretics (water pills) to increase urination and rid the body of water. Although the scale registers a lower number, this is only due to temporary dehydration, not because real weight loss has occurred. Although diuretics are completely ineffective as a weight-loss tool, those who are "addicted" to lowering the number on the scale maintain the illusion they have succeeded in dropping pounds. The names of diuretics also contribute to the false reassurance of safety: Weight Loss Cleanse and Flush, Natural Bloat-Away, Nutrition Watershed Diuretic, Total Lean Waterex.

Water is vital for all physiological systems. The body must be sufficiently hydrated in order to function properly. Dehydration through diuretics can damage the kidneys, the heart, and ultimately can result in death.

The Treatment of Bulimia:
From Demons to Daylight

The treatment of bulimia is complex, because the patient needs to allow herself to partake of the "therapy meal" with the therapist. She must become comfortable taking in and "digesting" the emotional connection in the relationship. And she needs to integrate and "metabolize" the caring into her system to become nourished. Her impulse is to get rid of emotional support just as she does with food. She both seeks care and rejects care; she wishes to be close, she fears to be close.

If she (or he) is a victim of sexual abuse, as many bulimics are, she struggles with a deep internal mistrust about whether the therapist has a hidden agenda to manipulate or exploit her. Why wouldn't she be suspicious of a person in charge? (We will discuss the crisis of sexual abuse and eating disorders in chapter 7.)

Because I believe all eating disorders are emotional communications from our inner self, I try to help each person translate into "feeling language" what her eating disorder is trying to express. I will ask a patient, "If your fat could talk, what would it say?" or "If your vomit could talk, what would it say and to whom?" "What is *your* theory about why you have this eating disorder?" Or I will ask, "When we help your eating problem get better, what is the very next issue that will come up for you?" With these questions, we try to form a partnership to discover the creative meaning of the eating problem.

The goal for eating disorder sufferers is to reclaim the self-expression they have detoured through their destructive behavior—to use their mouths for speaking their inner truth and not for bingeing and purging.

An effective therapy, such as the cases of Fran, Charlene, Gloria, and to some extent Megan, involves understanding how the person learned that her needs were bad and how she resorted to bulimia as her substitute for vital nourishment and nurturance. Behavioral and cognitive techniques to help her strategize alternatives to the binge/ purge cycle are crucial. Often medication for depression and anxiety is beneficial. Family and group therapy can also be valuable.[16]

And hopefully, eventually, the person, who once upon a time was derailed and muted by bulimia, will emerge with a full-bodied, expressive self, a self of vibrant and lusty dimension, filled with aliveness and passion.

Exercise Bulimia: "Addicted to Sweat"

A neighbor of mine challenged her overweight husband to lose weight, so she bought him an exercise CD. He responded cheerfully, "Great! I'll listen to it in the car as I drive to work!" We all had a good laugh at the lengths he went to avoid exercise.

Americans have a complicated relationship with exercise. Mark Twain once declared, "Whenever I feel the urge to exercise come on, I lie down until it passes." This comment is echoed by Lucy, of the comic strip *Peanuts,* "Exercise is a dirty word. Every time I hear it, I wash my mouth out with chocolate."

We are amused by these remarks because we all recognize that avoiding exercise is not healthy and that daily exercise benefits us greatly. We burn calories, discharge stress, improve our circulation, and lower our blood pressure; we sleep better and feel a sense of well-being from challenging our bodies.

So we ask ourselves: If some exercise is good, shouldn't more exercise be better? Not necessarily. Sometimes exercise becomes too much of a good thing. Instead of being a supportive friend, it becomes a hurtful enemy.[17]

Erica represents the opposite side of the coin from healthy exercise. Erica sets her alarm for 5:30 a.m. to go out running before school. She plays tennis five days a week, takes spin classes, and works out on her treadmill most nights. Erica cannot stop exercising even when she is tired or sick. Her mantra has adamantly become "no pain, no gain."

Erica is one of a growing number of people who have developed exercise addiction, an alternate form of bulimia. Because we hold exercise in such high esteem, we admire and envy those who devote great amounts of time to working out. Keeping fit and playing sports have become a national pastime, and we often don't necessarily realize when we, or someone we care about, are out of control with exercise. After all, exercise doesn't look like an eating disorder.

Many terms describe behavior like Erica's: compulsive exercise, exercise bulimia, exercise abuse, exercise addiction. Exercise is considered excessive when:

It significantly interferes with important activities. Erica often skipped family parties because she had to go to the gym or cancelled plans with friends in order to finish her workout routine. Erica arranged her life to accommodate her inner compulsive demand to exercise.

It occurs at inappropriate times. In the throes of her addiction, Erica exercised late into the night with her bedroom light turned off. While her family slept, she was secretly doing crunches.

It occurs in inappropriate settings. Connie, another exercise bulimic, ran in a New York City park before sunrise while it was still dark. Her drive to exercise trumped her need for caution.

The person exercises despite injury or other medical complications. Jeff had developed a stress fracture from jogging but continued despite increasing pain. Stacey developed a painful tennis elbow but was compelled to keep on playing.

Guilt, anxiety, or depression occurs if a workout is missed. Exercise addicts use exercise to deal with unhappy moods, such as depression or anxiety. They experience guilt and unease if unable to perform their exercise ritual.

The person does not take time to rest or recover between workouts.

The driving compulsion to keep exercising prevents the person from moderating his or her routine to allow the body a chance to recuperate.

A person does not permit him or herself to eat until the workout is accomplished. "I only allow myself to eat once I finish seven miles on the treadmill," states Natalie.

Compulsive exercise has little to do with the pleasure of movement and health. Its roots lie in struggles with self-esteem, perfectionism, fear, and control. Marsha described an inner pressure to continue a strenuous jogging regime, despite having injured her knee. She had created this punishing routine for herself but, although it was wearing her out, she kept pushing herself. Unlike most exercise bulimics, who just want to practice their obsession and hide from others the extent of their workouts, Marsha was exhausted and came to therapy to figure out how to help herself.

During the course of her therapy, Marsha expressed a deep anxiety about her husband's impending death. She felt helpless to cure Wayne's cancer but, while jogging, she would have temporary relief from her worries about him. "I feel exhilarated when I'm jogging. It's like a high. But afterwards my body aches and I feel empty inside." As a teenager, Marsha worried about being fat and had gone on fasts and liquid diets, with a brief period of anorexia. We discovered that her early struggles began around the time her grandmother was dying. It was helpful for Marsha to see this pattern—the loss of someone she loved made her reach for something to take away her pain and powerlessness. Focusing on dieting or fat or calories or weight or exercise presented a temporary sense of control over painful situations.

In the course of her therapy, Marsha began to feel worse. As she listened to her fatigue and cut down her workouts, she missed the escape from her fears that jogging provided. She became more depressed, as she no longer could hide from her suffering. Often patients will leave therapy at this point in an attempt to avoid facing their anguish directly. But Marsha did not "run away." We helped her through anticipatory mourning about Wayne's looming death. We also untangled some guilt feelings about her grandmother's death that she had never confronted. Although Marsha felt worse before she felt better, she concluded, "Having the courage to face my inner demons actually made me stronger. My hurtful, obsessive need to develop strong muscles diminished when I felt stronger emotionally to speak of my fear and pain in therapy and then to confide more in my husband. Wayne and I are now confronting his death together."

Coerced to Exercise

Two of my eating disorder patients—one bulimic, one a compulsive binge eater—had fathers who were Olympic medal winners in different sports. Heidi, bulimic and an exercise addict, described the pressure of growing up with a professional athlete father. "He ran our house like a military training camp and expected us to have the same enthusiasm for sports that he did. My mother had been a professional ice skater in Europe, so they were both of the belief that Sports is Our Family Religion. My natural inclination since I was a child is reading and riding my bike through the park. My parents found my choices laughable and not 'hard core' enough to fit in with our family values of an intense commitment to sports. They insisted I become involved in the school volleyball club, and the more discipline and dedication I showed, the more they praised me. And the more my real self got buried.

"I had tremendous shame about hating exercise and sports and competition. I believed there was something wrong with me since I *should* be the type of person who loves volleyball. But to avoid their ridicule, I bent over backward to prove I was worthy of their admiration. I was living a lie by pretending the volleyball team was the center of my life. In secret I vomited up all the resentment I felt at being coerced. I felt unlovable for my real self and just kept working harder and harder at my sport."

Heidi continued, "And then, one afternoon, jumping for the ball, I fell and broke my wrist. This put me out of commission, and for the first time I was justified taking time off. When I healed, my parents expected me to return to the team. I was a good girl and did what was expected while secretly vomiting up my food behind closed doors. Only after breaking my wrist a second time did my parents allow me to quit. My biggest shameful personal secret is how happy I was each time I broke my wrist. Did I do anything to contribute to breaking my wrist 'accidentally on purpose?' I can't say for sure, but I did have satisfaction that they couldn't blame me for not going back to volleyball."

The bulimic often creates a "false self" to please her parents and provide them with what she hopes will make them love her more. Her genuine self goes underground with her protest emerging only through vomiting. "If you can fake sincerity, you've got it made," Heidi ruefully quipped.

In her therapy, Heidi realized she felt like the tool in her family to bolster her parents' self-esteem and to help present the image they were the happy, healthy, all-American family. She felt disloyal for having separate wishes and needs and also angry at her parents for not seeing through her false gaiety around sports. Heidi expressed much shame, guilt, and anger before eventually unearthing the inner strength to return to her first loves of reading and bike riding.

Neil's parents called him "pudgy" as a child. They regulated his food, but he would retaliate by bingeing in secret rebellion. As he continued gaining weight, his parents coerced him to exercise. A vicious cycle was put into play: The more his parents restricted his food, the more Neil furtively overate. They then reacted by forcing him to exercise more. Neil described, "If we were stuck on the parkway in a traffic jam, my father would pull the car over to the right lane and make me get out of the car. I would be required to jog along the grassy edge of the parkway to get in some extra exercise until the traffic picked up speed, and my parents would drive to pick me up. I felt like a lonely orphan on these highway exiles. My rage at my father for expecting me not to waste a moment of potential exercise time made me enjoy bingeing even more behind his back. It was my revenge. But I also hurt myself as I continued gaining weight. I sacrificed myself to piss my parents off."

Realigning Your Exercise Patterns

Realigning your exercise patterns to break the addiction cycle means:

Reclaiming your pleasure in exercise.

Minimizing the inner conversation of your harsh conscience dictating what you should do. Speak back to that conscience, "Easy does it. Tomorrow is another day; I don't have to kill myself today."

Cultivating a relationship with your body in which you listen to when you are hungry, tired, worn out, or in pain. There is a fine line between exercise rejuvenating the body and depleting it. Your body speaks; listen carefully to become more aware of the messages. Every day is different. Some days you have more energy than others. Some days you need to go slowly or rest. You do not have to progressively compete with what you did the day before or set higher standards at each workout. Learn to evaluate when "enough is enough."

Ask yourself whether you are fearful of being still and at rest. What thoughts and feelings emerge if you are not able to exercise? Ross realized that intrusive thoughts about the sexual abuse by his grandfather arose every time he decided not to work out for a period of time. When we identified that Ross was suffering from post-traumatic stress disorder, his fear of stillness began to make more sense to him.

Reconnect with the fun of playing from when you were a child, before exercise got so serious. Heidi went back to her bike riding. Erica spent the summer months playing hopscotch with her daughter. My childhood friend, Carolyn, and I bought lots of rubber bands, looping them around our ankles to play Chinese jump rope just like when we were ten years old.

Food for Thought: Do You Exercise Compulsively?

If you are concerned that you may exercise too much, how you would answer the following questions:

> Do you pressure yourself to exercise more if you overeat?
> Did your interest in exercise begin with a desire to lose weight?
> Do you fear you will gain weight if you don't exercise every day?
> Are you preoccupied with being thinner and achieving a lower body mass/lean muscle ratio, as athletes do?
> Do you ever vomit, take laxatives, or diuretics after eating?
> Do you feel virtuous and self-righteous when dieting, restricting your dietary intake, or exercising?
> Do others express concern that you exercise too much?

Based on your answers, decide if your relationship with exercise is hurting you. It is important to see a health professional, such as a doctor, therapist, trainer, or nutritionist. Many compulsive exercisers find they need therapy to help them deal with exercise bulimia. Like Marsha, you may feel stronger after tackling your emotional problems directly rather than trying to exercise them away.

Binge Eating Disorder: Searching for Fullness

"I assault myself with food," states Celeste, describing her binge eating disorder in our first session.

"Why do you call it an assault?" I ask.

"I feel like I'm forcing food down my throat—food I don't even want and sometimes don't even like. It almost feels violent."

"And why do you require this violent assault with food?" I wonder.

"This is going to sound crazy, but I've done a lot of thinking about my bingeing. You should know that I've binged on and off at different points in my life. But it got worse after my mother died. I've gained a lot of weight since her death, and the bingeing has taken on a life of its own. That's why I decided to come for therapy now. It's all about my mother's death. I am furious at her for leaving me. When I binge, I feel like I'm beating my mother up for dying and abandoning me. Here's the crazy part: when I attack myself with food, it's like I attack her. A temper tantrum erupts inside of me and I tear into food. Mostly I gorge at night when I miss my mother the most."

"I can see you are angry about her dying, but why does that mean you have to beat yourself up?"

"Well," Celeste asks, "who else should I take it out on? There's nobody else to blame."

"But what are you to blame for? Is your bingeing a punishment for something?"

"I could have been a better daughter. I feel guilty. In her old age, my mother became progressively deaf, but I didn't get her help soon enough. The deafness made her more isolated than she had to be. I also became very impatient with her toward the end. I wasn't always that nice."

"So you were a human daughter, not a perfect daughter," I ventured.

"Actually, she wasn't always that nice to me either," admitted Celeste. "She could be critical and impatient and demanding."

"So she was a human mother, not a perfect mother."

Celeste begins to cry, "And now that she's dead, I can never try to make our relationship perfect anymore."

"You're right. You can't. Although I'm not sure mothers and daughters can ever make their relationship perfect. Whatever perfect means," I reply. "Celeste, you have a lot of grief, understandably so, about your mother's death. Let's talk more about your feelings and memories about her and figure out how to untangle your emotions from your eating."

Celeste welcomed the opportunity to speak in depth about her mother: Her mother's early, sad history; their times of deep loving connection; their times of anger and misunderstandings; Celeste's self-blame; and her reproaches of her mother as well. As Celeste spoke about her shortcomings as a daughter, she attacked herself with *words;* as she spoke about her mother's shortcomings, she attacked her mother with *words*. Rather than detouring her feelings through food, she was using her mouth for speaking, not for overeating. Celeste went on to explain the complicated, yet devoted, relationship she had with her mother.

After "chewing" over and "digesting" many memories about her mother over a course of time, Celeste suggested in one of her sessions, "I need to have a nighttime ritual to put myself to bed instead of bingeing. I remember a lullaby my mother used to sing to me when I was little. I have decided to sing it to myself each night as a way of evoking her loving spirit and breaking my attack with food. I want to sing it for you.

> *Sleep, baby, sleep,*
> *Your father is watching the sheep.*
> *Your mother is shaking the dreamland tree*
> *And down will fall a dream for thee*
> *Sleep, baby, sleep.*
> *Sleep, baby, sleep,*
> *The big stars are the sheep.*
> *The little ones are the lambs, I guess,*
> *The gentle moon is the shepherdess*
> *Sleep, baby, sleep.*
> *Sleep, baby, sleep.*

Celeste cried as she sang this song. I got teary too, picturing the tenderness of her mother singing this lullaby to her little girl. In her next session, Celeste said, "I seem to have interrupted the cycle of stuffing myself before going to bed. One morning when I awoke, my lashes and pillow were wet and I knew I had been crying in my sleep. I guess this must be another layer of grief emerging now that I'm not burying it with food."

Celeste's evening binge attacks eventually receded as she relived and accepted and integrated the tumultuous, yet loving, relationship she had with her mother.

In therapy, rarely does one insight or one interpretation or one breakthrough or one lullaby heal an eating disorder. It is only by summoning memories and buried emotions and bringing them into awareness that we gain different perspectives and possibilities of change. This awareness is like sunlight filtering through a stained glass window, illuminating different facets of the whole mosaic.

The Diagnosis of Binge Eating Disorder

In 2013, the fifth edition of the American Psychiatric Association's Diagnostic and Statistical Manual of Mental Disorders (*DSM-5*) finally included what we clinicians in the field of eating disorders already knew: Binge eating disorder is a valid and legitimate diagnosis. Although bulimia and anorexia have been listed in the *DSM*, it took this long for binge eating disorder—the most frequent eating disorder for both men and women—to be included.[18]

Binge eaters come in all shapes and sizes. Many large people are not binge eaters, while many average size people do struggle with compulsive eating problems. Not all obese people binge eat. Obesity describes someone's weight, binge eating describes someone's behavior.

Triggers for Binge Eating

For the binge eater, food is a drug that can soothe, comfort, relieve tension, blunt feelings, and even punish. Food is the safest, most legal, cheapest, most available mood-altering drug on the market.

The triggers that cause people to overeat emotionally when not physically hungry are varied:

Loneliness—using food to keep yourself company. Intense emptiness and isolation from others makes loneliness one of the most painful emotions. You can feel lonely even among other people.

Marjorie, a high school student, felt lonely every afternoon when she came home from school. Her mother worked late hours, and Marjorie sought "mothering" in the refrigerator.

Boredom—filling up empty time by bingeing. Boredom is a type of tension, not an absence of tension.

Carlos would compulsively arrange activities and social engagements for himself, but whenever he had time alone, he felt bored, tense, and uncomfortable. "I have no idea what I'm supposed to do with myself," he complained and resorted to overeating to fill up the empty, boring time until his next scheduled activity.

Depression—seeking comfort, companionship, or a heightened mood through overeating.

Following the death of his wife, Brent turned to binge eating to quell his pain. He was depressed both at the loss of his wife and at the conviction his life was over now that she was dead.

Preventive bingeing—overeating to prevent yourself from being hungry at some future time.

Brianna was a saleswoman who drove to meetings throughout the city. Unsure how long each meeting would last and whether she might get hungry and not have a chance to eat, Brianna compulsively over-ate in her car to prevent possible future hunger.

Anesthesia—using food to put yourself to sleep or to numb yourself.

Ben was the victim of a violent mugging and suffered flashbacks and insomnia. Gorging on food helped make him sleepy and sedated.

Transitions—bingeing between activities to help you switch gears.

Leah, a single mother, arrived home from work and then her children came home from school. Her evenings involved helping the children with homework, making dinner, bathing, and putting the kids to sleep. She ate throughout the afternoon, trying to fortify herself for the long night ahead of chores and child care and responsibilities.

Fatigue—overeating to refuel yourself rather than resting, napping, or sleeping when tired.

Scott would pump himself up between his day job and his night job through compulsive eating. Not able to respond to his body's need for rest, he attempted to use bingeing to boost his energy.

Lack of structure—using emotional eating to replace the missing structure of the work week, such as at night, on weekends, or on vacation.

Rita thrived on her hurried, demanding schedule as an emergency room nurse. When she had days off from the hospital, she felt at a loss without the hectic schedule and manically ate large portions of food to fill in the blanks of free, unstructured time.

Separation/abandonment—using a connection with food to avoid feeling the pain of rejection or the loss of a loved one.

Ashley struggled with leaving home to an out-of-town college and deeply missed her friends and family back home. She overate nightly with the food she brought into her dorm in an attempt to recreate a comforting connection to her family and the dinners they ate together every evening.

Procrastination—using emotional eating to avoid or postpone the anxiety of some dreaded task.

Frank was a freshman in college, but often felt inadequate to the tasks at hand. His evenings were spent bingeing over the sink in order to avoid the anxiety of getting down to his homework and confronting his uncertainty over whether he was truly "college material."

Fear of crying—overeating to avoid crying because it feels too painful or too indulgent or because you worry that once you start, you'll never stop.

Jane had been blindsided by her husband's request for a divorce at the same time her mother was undergoing treatment for breast cancer. Needing to "stay strong," Jane buried her sorrow and tears through her eating binges.

Avoidance of sexual intimacy—overeating as a substitute for sex or a way to avoid sex.

Donna was uneasy with sex. She avoided her husband by stalling her bedtime and, instead, would stuff herself in the kitchen pantry.

Anger—biting or stuffing food to discharge angry feelings.

Craig was passed over for a promotion at his office. He discharged his anger at his boss through nighttime overeating, with much hostile biting and chewing.

Resentment—"swallowing" resentments and detouring them through emotional eating rather than confronting them directly.

Tanya felt strong resentment that her boyfriend of three years was not broaching the subject of marriage. Wanting to avoid conflict and afraid of alienating him, she buried her resentment in binge eating.

Guilt/shame—attempting to alleviate and punish oneself for guilty feelings through overeating.

After his father died, Dennis grew remorseful and guilty for not having visited him more frequently in the nursing home. He turned to food, his "substance of choice," to distract himself from this gnawing self-blame.

Disappointment/rejection—using food to "make it up to yourself" for feeling deprived.

Faith was rejected from the business administration program she hoped to attend and tried to lessen the pain of disappointment with the temporary solace of food.

Chronic physical pain—overeating as an attempt to soothe yourself to feel better.

Nelly suffered from arthritis of the back and, when the pain flared up, her eating disorder also flared as she attempted to "medicate" her pain with food.

Overwhelmed—having too much responsibility on your "plate" and seeking an oasis in food.

Kimberly worked full-time, had two children at home, was caring for an aging father, and also involved in a master's program. Food became her oasis in the midst of overwhelm.

Envy—feelings of greed, jealousy, and envy can be so painful that people turn to food to camouflage their feelings of deprivation.

When Brooke discovered her best friend was pregnant, she was filled with envy and shame. She had been struggling with infertility and could not bear to face her friend's pregnancy. A steady regime of bingeing "helped" her swallow these unacceptable feelings, as well as making her belly feel big and full.

Anticipatory grief—preparing for the death of a loved one, or a dreaded move, or a medical procedure by padding yourself with excess food to "dial down" the fear.

Alma's sister was declining from Alzheimer's disease and, to cushion herself against her sister's loss, Alma found herself bingeing incessantly.

"Hangry"—a double whammy trigger combining hunger and anger.

Irene coined this term to describe the two ingredients that consistently led her to overeat.

Dieting—the most common trigger for binge eating when the deprivation caused by the diet invariably becomes unbearable.

Olivia found herself on an ongoing diet and binge cycle every time she tried to follow a rigid, diet plan. Breakthrough bingeing would assert itself as her unsatisfied body rebelled.

Stress and Compulsive Overeating

People experience stress when they cannot cope with the demands in their life and the strain and pressure feels overwhelming. Most often, stress is brought on by complications involving relationships, health, work, school, money. Stress can be experienced either emotionally (anxiety, irritability, nervousness) or physically (exhaustion, insomnia, muscle tension, stomach problems, high blood pressure).

People vary considerably in their capacity to handle stress. Some soldiers return from war relatively intact emotionally, while others in the same unit—who have been through the same events—may develop post-traumatic stress disorder. The *internal* experience of an event, unique to each person, can be perceived as either neutral, benign, or a stressful threat.

For some people, stress can at times be beneficial because it stimulates motivation, ambition, and the energy to get through demanding times. But stress can also lead to chronic worry, which burns people out and, in turn, can lead to emotional eating.

The tension and crunch of daily hassles, *microstressors,* sometimes have an even greater negative impact on a person's health than more acute, traumatic stressors that generally have a beginning and end point. Microstressors are those chronic thorns-in-the-side experiences: traffic jams, conflicts with neighbors, nightly barking dogs, stalled subways, irritable bosses. These are not major catastrophes, but they stir up a gnawing anxiety and helplessness. To relieve that strain, the binge eater turns to the comfort of food.

Stress Scale for Adults

In 1967, psychiatrists Thomas Holmes and Richard Rahe examined the medical records of over 5,000 patients to determine whether stressful events might cause illness. Holmes and Rahe asked people to examine the changes, losses, and transitions in their lives over the previous 12 months and to tally a list of 43 life events. A number from 11 to 100 was assigned to each event depending on the severity of the change. "Major changes in a person's life have effects that carry over for long periods of time. It is like dropping a rock into a pond. After the initial splash, the ripples of stress may continue in your life for at least a year," they explain.

Since that initial study in 1967, further research and clinical evidence validates the close connection between stress and illness—and binge eating, I would add.

The Holmes–Rahe Stress Inventory Scale

Life event	*Life change units*
Death of a spouse	100
Divorce	73
Marital separation	65
Imprisonment	63
Death of a close family member	63
Personal injury or illness	53
Marriage	50
Dismissal from work	47
Marital reconciliation	45
Retirement	45
Change in health of family member	44
Pregnancy	40
Sexual difficulties	39
Gain a new family member	39
Business readjustment	39
Change in financial state	38
Death of a close friend	37
Change to different line of work	36
Change in frequency of arguments	35
Major mortgage	32
Foreclosure of mortgage or loan	30
Change in responsibilities at work	29
Child leaving home	29
Trouble with in-laws	29
Outstanding personal achievement	28
Spouse starts or stops work	26
Begin or end school	26
Change in living conditions	25
Revision of personal habits	24

Trouble with boss	23
Change in working hours or conditions	20
Change in residence	20
Change in schools	20
Change in recreation	19
Change in religious activities	19
Change in social activities	18
Minor mortgage or loan	17
Change in sleeping habits	16
Change in number of family reunions	15
Change in eating habits	15
Vacation	13
Christmas	12
Minor violation of law	11

Source: T.H. Holmes and R.H. Rahe, "The Social Readjustment Rating Scale," Journal of Psychosomatic Research, 1967, vol. 11, 213–218.

I would include in this list additional stressors, such as the anniversary of a loved one's death, stopping smoking, experiencing a natural disaster such as hurricane Katrina or Sandy, a family member serving in the military, having to give up driving because of age or health reasons, and the death of a beloved pet.

A version of the stress scale, designed for adolescents, includes death/divorce/remarriage of a parent, breakup with a girlfriend or boyfriend, failure in school, death/illness of friend or sibling, change in acceptance by peers, becoming involved with drugs or alcohol, and change in parents' finances.

According to Holmes and Rahe, if you have experienced total stress within the last 12 months of 250 units or greater, you may be overstressed. Persons with a lower stress tolerance may be overstressed at levels of 150.

No current research confirms the connection between the stress scale and eating disorders. However, I think this inventory leads us to a deeper appreciation of how major events in a person's life can provoke a heightened search for comfort through binge eating. It is noteworthy that even good life events can cause stress.

Diets Do Work . . . Until They Don't

The original meaning of the word "diet" came from the Latin (diaeta) and meant "way of life." The current meaning of diet implies restriction, deprivation, constraint, and limitation.

Binge eaters turn to diets in the hope of getting their overeating under control, to provide a structure of what they should eat, and to lose weight. Every month of every year, diet books feature prominently on the bestseller lists. They dictate what we should eat, what we shouldn't eat, how much we should eat, and even when. Some diets count calories, some count points, some consist of only liquids, some provide processed foods, some eliminate certain foods, some go by your blood type. There is a diet for every letter of the alphabet from Atkins, to Blood Type diet, to Cabbage diet, to Detox diets, Elimination diet, Fit for Life . . . to Vegan, Weight Watchers, and the Zone! And if choosing gets too complicated, you can always resort to the Breatharian diet in which no food is consumed, based on the belief that food is not necessary for human subsistence.[19]

In her therapy session, April reviewed all the restrictive diets she had submitted herself to over the years. At different points over the years her list included:

no canned food	no gluten	no whey
no milk	no meat	no eggs
low glycemic index foods	no casein	no lactose
no sugar	no artificial sweeteners	only organic
no oil	no preservatives, no MSG	no white rice

no eating fruits after protein	no combining protein + carbs	no yeast
no water with meals	water before meals	no white flour
no peanut butter	no added salt	no cookies
no sautéed food	no high-carb veggies	no candy
no sugary fruit	no bread	no honey
fiber in every meal	nothing fried	no ice cream
no eating before bedtime		

April described preparing low-calorie hamburgers out of marinated tofu, pasta out of spaghetti squash, and baking chocolate chip cookies out of mashed white beans!

Through her therapy, April realized her obsessive dieting was not working to help her lose weight, become healthier, or achieve inner peace of mind. April finally concluded: "In order not to binge, I must permit myself to eat what I want to eat. The bottom line is tofu is not hamburgers, squash is not spaghetti, and white beans are definitely not chocolate chip cookies. I am tired of 'outsourcing' my eating to a diet—someone else's rules and regulations. I am now on the path of transitioning from Outsourcing to Ownership!"

In addition to the *emotional* deprivation that diets cause, the *physiological* consequences of dieting are also detrimental. Diets lower a person's metabolism and the repetitive weight loss/gain cycle leads to an ever-greater accumulation of body fat. *Why Women Need Chocolate*, a book with a most beguiling title, states, "Dieting causes brain turbulence. It decreases your brain chemicals and brain sugar supplies, increases your food cravings, and depresses your mood."

Dieting decreases your serotonin level which is necessary for stabilizing your mood and maintaining a sense of calm. The body reacts to this serotonin depletion by craving carbohydrates. The dieter once again attributes her break through bingeing as a *personal failure*, rather than as a *biological response* to her restriction and deprivation.[20]

Diets will always be seductive to binge eaters because they do work. But *only temporarily.* While diets attempt to *externally* fix, regulate, and control eating behavior, they do not resolve the *inner* emotional hunger that continues to provoke the bingeing—the hunger from the heart, not the stomach. No matter how many foods we banish or calories we count, dieting colludes with our fear of tackling the emotional heartbeat of what promotes our disordered eating—the hunger of our soul, the hunger to feel a vital connection to our desires and needs, the hunger to feel alive in our own skin.

All true healing must begin with the human heart.

We live in a culture that does not encourage the full expression of emotions and exhorts us, "If you don't have anything good to say, don't say anything." "Suck it up." "Don't make a mountain out of a molehill." "You're too sensitive." "Shame on you!" "Grin and bear it." "Get over yourself." "Smile and the world smiles with you, cry and you cry alone." "Keep a stiff upper lip." "Just forgive and forget." And as the songs go, "Accentuate the positive, eliminate the negative, and don't mess with Mr. In-Between!" "Smile, though your heart is breaking," "When you walk through a storm keep your head up high," "Put on a happy face," and, "Don't worry, be happy. Every little thing is gonna be all right."

Binge eaters are often ashamed or guilty about what they feel. They worry that by confronting their emotions they will be overwhelmed by them. In fact, it is not our feelings that cause binge eating. *It is our attempt not to feel our feelings.*

Such was the case of Evelyn.

Evelyn returned to binge eating when her husband announced his upcoming retirement. Evelyn acted delighted that Larry would achieve his long-cherished wish of leaving his banking job. But she secretly worried about the changes his retirement might cause to her own life. She felt guilty and ashamed by her ungenerous reaction. Overeating diverted her away from her "selfishness," but, of course, it resolved nothing.

In therapy, Evelyn came to realize how her own retirement the previous year was the first time she ever enjoyed private time just for herself. Coming from a family of eight children and raising her own family of five while working full-time gave Evelyn little chance to have private time and discover her own interests. Larry's retirement felt threatening to her new-found freedom. "He will be underfoot," said Evelyn morosely. "I will have to cook for him and not be free to just do my own thing." As Evelyn came to appreciate the valuable meaning of loving her own personal time and space, she felt less ashamed to discuss with her husband how they would negotiate this new chapter together.

The awareness of the emotions aggravating her bingeing became our gateway to better understand Evelyn's inner self. We helped Evelyn focus on what she *was* feeling, not what she *should* be feeling. The key ingredient in resolving binge eating, as Evelyn discovered, is to embrace and accept our feelings, learn to honor them, digest them, integrate them, and communicate them unapologetically.

A Tour Guide to Feelings

When we automatically translate all our emotions, needs, and hungers as cravings for food, we never devote our attention to what is truly bothering us. We shortchange ourselves from knowing our true feelings and thus from attaining true nourishment.

Be curious about what you are feeling, rather than judgmental.

Feelings are not facts. Although Evelyn felt conflicted about Larry's retirement, she did nothing to sabotage him and, therefore, had nothing realistically to feel guilty about. All feelings have a beginning, middle and an end. You will not be stuck forever feeling uncomfortable.

Feelings do pass *whether or not you eat over them!*

All human beings have a variety of feelings from generous to unkind and selfish. That's human beings for you!

To cope with feelings, we need to (1) name them, (2) claim them, and (3) aim them. Aiming them *inwardly* means cultivating an inner self-acceptance of all we feel, while aiming them *outwardly* involves communicating and expressing ourselves directly to others. Or, said another way about feelings: We need to face them, trace them, embrace them!

No one is so unique that their feelings are necessarily worthy of shame and self-hatred. As the Roman philosopher Terence declared on the universality of feelings, "I am human. Let nothing human be alien to me." And then there's pop singer Bette Midler's philosophy of accepting emotions: "I always try to balance the light with the heavy—a few tears of human spirit in with the sequins and the fringes!"

A Tour Guide to Conscious Eating

The tour guide to "declaring peace with emotional eating" and resolving bingeing involves increasing our awareness and consciousness of the pace of our eating. So many of us eat automatically until the plate is empty. Or we eat quickly in order to consume as much food as possible. Or we heard as children, "When you finish your lima beans, *then* you can have dessert," which is a form of rewarding children for eating, regardless of their hunger or preferences.

Few children get the message to slow down, savor, relish, really taste, and take pleasure in their food. Helene, fed up with bingeing on cheap, chemical-laden diet ice cream that she didn't even particularly like, decided to treat herself to her favorite ice cream, a rare treat she had not permitted herself for years. At the store, she searched for mocha chip ice cream, but it was not to be found. Undeterred, she purchased a pint of coffee and a pint of mint chip, mixed them up at home, and sat down with the bowl, lovingly tasting each creamy spoonful. Helene closed her eyes the better to focus on the luscious flavors. Rather than bingeing on this "exotic" treat as she had feared, it filled her up with satisfaction. And when she had enough, she stopped. Knowing she could always give herself permission to provide this real, enjoyable food next time she wanted it made her not have to panic over this ice cream rendezvous with, "let me get it all in now before I take it away from myself again."

The concept of conscious or mindful eating can be a form of meditation. Just as there are meditations that involve sitting, breathing, standing, praying, chanting, or walking, eating can also be a way of meditating as well.[21]

Nibble slowly. Savor the flavor, texture, temperature, colors, fragrance, spices. You will experience your food more intensely and with more pleasure. *Pleasure,* not restriction or deprivation, is the ultimate antidote to binge eating!

Sink your teeth into life, not into excess food!

Obesity and Overweight: Is Fat Your Fate?

If shame could cure obesity, there wouldn't be a fat woman in the world.

—Susan Wooley, Ph.D.

"O-Beast is what I really deserve to be called rather than obese," Matthew says mournfully. "I eat like a beast and then I feel like one for being so fat."

Matthew is not alone. His rueful comment expresses the isolation, despair, and humiliation so many obese and overweight people feel.

Overweight and obesity have become a high-profile topic in the media. Headlines blare what we already know to be true: Americans are fat and getting fatter.[22]

Recent headlines include:

"Overweight Adolescents Have Tripled Since 1980"

"World Health Organization Turns Attention to Obesity"

"Another Study Finds a Link Between Excess Weight and Cancer"
"Risk of Birth Defects is Linked to Obesity"
"Obesity Among Children in the U.S. Has Reached Epidemic Proportions"
"Overweight Increases the Risk of Alzheimer's"
"75 Percent of Americans Will Be Overweight by 2020"
"Disturbing Diabetes Forecast Linked to Obesity"

Determining Obesity

The body mass index (BMI) is a formula that calculates the ratio of a person's weight to height. It has been the medical profession's standard measurement of overweight and obesity for decades.

To figure out your own BMI, plug your numbers into this formula:

Calculate your height in inches and square it (multiply it by itself). For example, Debra, a 5'4" woman, would multiply 64 inches times 64 for a total of 4,096.

Divide your weight by the height number you calculated above. Debra weighs 175 pounds, so she would divide 175 by 4,096. The result is .04.

Take that result and multiply it by 703. Debra's body mass index is 30.0.

Here's what your BMI number means:

Underweight: your BMI is less than 18.5
Normal: 18.5to 24.9
Overweight: 25 to 29.9
Obese: 30 to 39.9
Morbid obesity (more than 100 pounds overweight): 40 and higher

According to her BMI, Debra is obese, but on the low end of the range. But what does this number really tell us about Debra? Can we truly evaluate her health, lifestyle, emotional resilience, nutritional levels, or fitness level on the basis of just one number?

The traditional BMI equation does have some flaws. Strong, fit men and women and athletes, with their heavy muscle mass, may measure obese on this rating system, but are actually within normal limits. Not all obese people have health problems or an increase in health risks, so measuring their obesity may be irrelevant. Weight carried on the hips and thighs (pear-shaped body) has been associated with a lower risk of cardiovascular disease. An obese person who is fit and eats healthfully can have a positive health profile regardless of BMI.

Another, perhaps more accurate, way to determine obesity is to measure your waist circumference. Your waist measurement correlates with abdominal fat; a larger waist is associated with a higher health risk. Men who have a waist circumference of 40 inches or more, and women who have a waist circumference of 35 inches or more, are considered to be at increased health risk.[23] However, here again, we are evaluating people's health based on one number.

Because not all obese individuals are at an increased health risk, and therefore may not necessarily require weight loss, the Edmonton Obesity Staging System was developed as a screening tool to determine risk factors. The system uses a five-stage classification to determine obesity-related risk factors. The stages range from 0 (obese with no health problems) to 4 (severe impairment). This system helps show that not all obese people have problematic health issues.[24]

Still another classification is the national Million Hearts initiative. The focus of this initiative to prevent heart attacks and strokes isn't weight loss. Instead, the program focuses on improving health behaviors. The focus is on the ABCS: appropriate aspirin therapy, blood pressure control, cholesterol, and smoking cessation.

Fat is not all bad. Having some fat on one's body is actually quite necessary. Fat insulates and protects our internal organs. Fat is a source of energy. Fat is needed for the production of hormones and for menstruation and fertility in women. Fat serves as padding if we fall![25]

The equation that thin = healthy and fat = unhealthy does not stand up to scrutiny. A woman of "ideal" BMI who lives on cigarettes, coffee, and fast food will not be as healthy as an overweight woman who works out regularly and eats healthfully.

Whether being overweight or obese impacts your health depends on a number of factors, including age, gender, fat distribution, and how physically active you are. If you are obese and surrounded by supportive people, you may not be as affected by society's negative judgments and better able to enjoy your life more fully. But if being fat hinders your health or self-esteem, it may lessen your enjoyment of life. Shame may cause you to not feel free in your own body, to avoid socializing, or making love, or going on vacation. Nick described his fatness as a "straitjacket" on his body and in his life.

Causes

Is obesity really about eating too many cookies and ice cream? Or being a couch potato? Overweight and obesity are complex conditions with multiple causes, and scientists are still trying to fathom all the components.

What we do know is obesity is not caused solely by our food choices, but also by:

Heredity. Your family's unique genetic makeup contributes to your predisposition to gain weight. Just as brown skin or tallness or blue eyes get passed down from parent to child, so does body type. Many people fail to lose weight or keep it off because their bodies are genetically programmed to be fat. Heredity also influences our metabolism (the rate we burn calories). Researchers estimate that 50 to 80 percent of our weight and metabolism is the result of genetics, and scientists have uncovered more than 50 genes that influence appetite and metabolism.[26] You can alter heredity only up to a point. To a large degree, heredity is destiny. It is nobody's fault.

Antoinette came from a family of obese parents and sisters. Their attitude about their family fatness was nonchalant, "It is what it is," and they took pleasure in sharing good times and good food together. Antoinette's fat was a non-issue for her and her family, and she communicated this unapologetically to the world. Antoinette married Hank, a thin, athletic man, who enjoyed the unconditional love Antoinette's family conveyed because it was so different from his own emotionally constricted background. He loved his wife's fat body enveloping him when they were in bed, "She's like a mermaid protecting me!" Hank laughed.

Age. As we get older, our metabolism slows down. Many patients describe with dismay how, once upon a time, as young adults, they could eat whatever they wanted without gaining weight. Particularly after menopause, women experience slower metabolism and unwanted weight gain.

Food choices. Eating a diet heavy in high-calorie, low-nutrition foods will pack on weight. The documentary film, *Super Size Me*, reveals how the restaurant industry has steadily increased the portions of fast food and take-out food. French fries, soda, hamburgers, chips, and other foods are now served in gargantuan portions. If we are oblivious, we pay the price in pounds.

Dieting. Most obese people have repeatedly dieted, with little lasting success. Often, they discover that restrictive dieting invariably causes a backlash of out-of-control eating that adds on even more weight. For every depriving diet, an opposite and equal binge is waiting on the horizon to strike. The lifelong cycle of dieting > weight loss > deprivation > weight gain, repeated over and over again, causes the metabolism to slow down and the body to resist further weight loss. Doctors often recommend remaining at a higher weight rather than yo-yoing up and down to avoid this metabolic shut-down and the resulting increase in the body's fat-to-muscle ratio. According to Dr. Rubin Andres of the National Institute on Aging, "A mild, gradual increase in weight over time may be the healthiest weight pattern and compatible with the longest life."[27]

Activity level. Exercise is the key ingredient in revving up metabolism. Our love affair with cars and labor-saving devices causes us to expend fewer calories than in past generations. A patient, Barbara, observed: "Today I drove to the avenue to get the newspaper and milk, I had the cleaning lady do the laundry and vacuum the house, I shopped for clothes on-line, and then watched television after dinner. I never realized how sedentary I've become. No wonder I've gained so much weight."

Psychological issues. Anxiety and depression may cause people to soothe themselves by overeating when they are not hungry. Binge eating disorder will cause people to gain weight.

Medications. Certain medications, including some antidepressants and drugs for bipolar disorder, can cause weight gain. Medications may contribute to weight gain by changing your satiety center so you do not realize you are eating more or by impeding your metabolism. Sometimes your doctor can substitute an alternative medication that is more weight neutral.

The Solution

Obesity may increase your risk for developing type 2 diabetes, high blood pressure, high cholesterol, heart disease, stroke, breathing problems, sleep apnea, and certain cancers. To manage or improve obesity, the goal should be enhancing your health and well-being through *more exercise, better eating, and self acceptance,* not through dieting down to some "ideal" weight that you will not be able to maintain over the long run.

Given how widespread and complex overweight and obesity are, controversy abounds as to the best approaches and solutions.

Weighing the Options: Finding Your Personal Path

Five different approaches can address the problems of overweight and obesity. There is no "one size fits all," so each obese person must discover what works uniquely for him or her.

Commercial Weight-Loss Programs

For many people, commercial weight-loss programs, with their structure, group meetings, weekly weigh-ins, and prepared food, offer beneficial support to promote healthier eating. Rather than battling their out-of-control eating all alone, people often welcome learning how to manage their eating while sharing with others in the same boat.

Adam explained how after his wife died of breast cancer, he gained 80 pounds in the following several years. "My life was so scrambled after Gina died, and my eating got completely messed up," Adam related. "Everything felt like hunger. My sadness felt like hunger, my loneliness felt like hunger, anger like hunger, even insomnia felt like hunger. So I ate and ate. In addition to therapy, where I really worked on separating out my grief from my hunger, I went to a program. The external structure helped me learn how to eat healthfully and cook for myself, something Gina had always done. I was so depleted that I really appreciated the support and being told what to eat until I could get myself back on track."

The key to success in a commercial weight-loss program is twofold: (1) not to turn the recommended eating plan into a restrictive diet that will eventually backfire and (2) being willing to follow the maintenance plan once weight loss is achieved. Alexa lost 65 pounds on the program she attended and assumed after all her hard work that she was immune from gaining the weight back. After denying for months how much she was overeating and slowly regaining, Alexa returned to her group to commit to their ongoing maintenance plan. Many obese people can possibly lose weight, but keeping it off is another matter, as it means making major lifestyle changes with ongoing vigilance.

National Association to Advance Fat Acceptance (NAAFA)

Founded in 1969, NAAFA is a national civil rights organization dedicated to improving the quality of life of fat people. NAAFA strives to eliminate discrimination based on body size and provides fat people with tools for self-empowerment through education, advocacy, and member support.

NAAFA champions the view that overweight or obesity is not a moral weakness nor a lack of willpower or even necessarily caused by overeating. Heredity and repeated dieting, which lowers metabolism, are possible causes of obesity. NAAFA also encourages people to make peace with their fat and to live more fulfilling lives without shame or defensiveness, regardless of what they weigh.

NAAFA asserts that people naturally come in all sizes and shapes. Just as we readily accept that people grow to different heights, so we need to accept people are a range of different weights as well. Some obese men and women have eating disorders, some do not: "People with eating disorders deserve effective treatment and are often able to recover; however, their weight may or may not change in that process. An arbitrarily chosen weight should not be a goal of treatment, since weight is not under direct control. The focus should be on a sustainable, high quality of life, and on helping the person to accept the resulting body size."[28]

NAAFA states that weight loss is not the solution for a fat person's emotional distress, since so much of that distress is due to fat discrimination. The solution is to address anti-fat prejudice and outlaw discrimination. NAAFA points out that you can be fat and fit.

Matthew, whom we met at the beginning of this section, blamed himself for the frequently insulting taunts people would make about his weight. He, like other fat people, had internalized the abusive comments which added to his low self-esteem and depression. By joining NAAFA, Matthew became part of a forceful community. This helped break through his shame and taught him to understand his obesity was not his fault.

Overeaters Anonymous

This program believes compulsive overeating is a progressive disease that affects a person physically, emotionally, and spiritually. Patterned on the principles of Alcoholics Anonymous, members acknowledge they are powerless over food, and overeating has made their life unmanageable. OA offers self-help support groups where members share their strength, hope, and experience; they choose a personal sponsor to guide them; and commit to the 12 steps of the program. OA promises that by practicing the program, the obsession to overeat will be lifted, but not cured. OA encourages striving for "progress, not perfection."[29]

The Twelve Steps are the heart of the OA recovery program:

1. We admitted we were powerless over food—that our lives had become unmanageable.
2. Came to believe that a power greater than ourselves could restore us to sanity.
3. Made a decision to turn our will and our lives over to the care of God as we understood Him.
4. Made a searching and fearless moral inventory of ourselves.
5. Admitted to God, to ourselves and to another human being the exact nature of our wrongs.
6. Were entirely ready to have God remove all these defects of character.
7. Humbly asked Him to remove our shortcomings.
8. Made a list of all persons we had harmed and became willing to make amends to them all.
9. Made direct amends to such people wherever possible, except when to do so would injure them or others.
10. Continued to take personal inventory and when we were wrong, promptly admitted it.
11. Sought through prayer and meditation to improve our conscious

contact with God as we understand Him, praying only for knowledge of His will for us and the power to carry that out.

12. Having had a spiritual awakening as the result of these Steps, we tried to carry this message to compulsive overeaters and to practice these principles in all our affairs.

The Serenity Prayer of OA teaches how to cope with life without compulsive overeating:

> *God grant me the Serenity to accept the things I cannot change,*
> *The courage to change the things I can,*
> *And the wisdom to know the difference.*

The Program offers slogans which have been described as "life wisdom written in shorthand:"

> My best friend, food, became my worst enemy.
> The overeater is described as "I want what I want when I want it."
> Abstinence from compulsive overeating is a journey, not a destination.
> Change is a process, not an event.
> Easy does it.
> Wear life like a loose-fitting garment.
> First things first.
> Live and let live.
> One day at time.
> Let go and let God.
> Keep It Simple.
> This, too, shall pass. Stress does not last forever.
> Live in the NOW.
> The OA program is for those who are sick and tired of being sick and tired.

Practice HALT, meaning Don't get too Hungry, Angry, Lonely or Tired.

I can do something for 24 hours—avoid compulsive overeating—which would appall me if I thought I had to keep it up for a lifetime.

Just for today I will try to live through this day only and not tackle my whole life problems at once.

One compulsive bite is too many, a thousand is not enough.

Insanity is defined as eating the same way over and over again, expecting different results.

Compulsive overeaters have a *living* problem, not an eating problem.

Bariatric Surgery

Weight-loss (bariatric) surgery is a procedure designed to make the stomach smaller, which in turn limits the amount of food a person can ingest. As a result, people feel physically full much sooner, usually leading them to eat less and lose weight. The American Society for Metabolic and Bariatric Surgery (ASMBS) claims, "Surgical treatment is medically necessary because it is the only proven method of achieving long-term weight control for the morbidly obese." Their web site offers testimonials and dramatic before/after pictures of people whose lives were enhanced by surgery. Patients describe their new-found joy in walking without getting out of breath, wearing a bathing suit, making love with more ease, fitting into an airline or movie seat.

Bariatric surgery may improve medical conditions related to obesity such as reflux, heart disease, sleep apnea, type 2 diabetes, and possibly enhance a woman's fertility through improved blood sugar and hormone levels. According to the American Society for Bariatric Surgery, whatever risks are involved with the surgery should be viewed in the larger context that severe obesity is a chronic, frequently progressive, life-threatening disease that requires drastic measures.[30]

Doctors recommend that people considering bariatric surgery should meet these guidelines:

1. Have a body mass index (BMI) of 40 or more.
2. Have a life-threatening or disabling condition worsened by their weight (BMI of at least 35).
3. Have been obese for at least five years.
4. Have no history of alcohol abuse.
5. Have no history of depression or any major emotional disorder.
6. Be between 18 and 65 years of age.

Weight-loss surgery has gained popularity as people despair of solving their obesity problem on their own. There are several types of bariatric surgery, including gastric bypass, sleeve gastrectomy, and laparoscopic adjustable gastric banding, or lap band. In the lap band procedure, a small band containing an inflatable balloon is placed around the upper part of the stomach, creating a small pouch. The doctor can tighten or loosen the band according to a person's individual weight loss needs.

Robert came for therapy following his bariatric surgery. He wanted guidance on handling his son's compulsive eating and obesity. Robert felt guilty that he was to blame for being a bad role model during Bobby's childhood and did not want his son to suffer with his weight the way Robert had.

In our initial consultation, Robert began by first sharing his successful experience with bariatric surgery.

Mary Anne: What made you finally decide to go for bariatric surgery?

Robert: I needed three different surgeries to close a hiatal incisional hernia resulting from a kidney surgery and none of them worked because I was obese. I decided on bariatric surgery because I had to lose a lot of weight quickly for this health reason. This was a life-or-death issue for my health, not a decision to lose weight to improve my appearance.

MA: What had you tried in the past to lose weight? Had anything ever been successful or helpful?

R: I tried many things in the past. I went on a liquid diet, lost 80 pounds, and gained 100 back. I went to two commercial weight-loss groups, had customized programs designed for me by nutritionists, tried just about every diet, ate only protein, took diet pills. Nothing worked in the long term.

MA: When you went for the surgery, would you consider yourself an overeater/a binge eater/an emotional eater? How would you describe your eating patterns?

R: I am genetically disposed to obesity, everyone on my mother's side is obese. I always overate and ate quickly. I was not a binger, but a steady snacker, a compulsive "wolfer-downer" of food, and always ate huge portions.

MA: What about now since the surgery?

R: I eat slowly with very small portions and lots of liquids. You really have no choice because your food comes up on you if you eat fast or a lot. Also, you can't drink quickly, you have to sip. Most nights I do treat myself to a whole pint of vanilla ice cream.

MA: How did you decide which surgery to go for—gastric bypass versus lap band?

R: I had the lap band because I wanted the choice to be reversible plus I wanted the option to have gradual tightening so I could progressively eat less and lose more weight. I also wanted the ability to have the band loosened if needed for medical reasons (operations, etc.) that require a post-operative regime of drinking lots of fluids.

MA: What was the maximum of weight you lost? How much weight loss have you maintained?

R: I was 285 when I had the lap band, and the maximum I lost was 80 pounds. I now have maintained a 60-pound weight loss for the past two and a half years. Occasionally I continue to lose a pound or two, but never gain. It took me less than a year to lose 60 pounds.

MA: What is the biggest benefit from the surgery?

R: Primarily the biggest benefits for me have been increased mobility, increased energy, increased libido, less knee pain, less overall pain, my hernia basically healed, and better overall health. I'm not so scared of the future and going into my later years with obesity-related illnesses. Secondly, I definitely have increased self-esteem, less food expenses, less eating out as a way of life. Now I can walk on the beach without being self-conscious and needing to cover up with a tee shirt. I can exercise without pain and without feeling obese every second of the day. I no longer have sleep apnea, so I sleep much better and don't snore anymore. My wife rejoices!

MA: Are there any down sides?

R: The biggest problem is throwing up when I eat too fast or when eating the wrong kinds of foods or choking for the same reasons. Eating is never fun or enjoyable any more, but rather a chore to ingest required nutrients. Social events where eating is the central activity are difficult for me. Also, I can feel the port for the band under my skin; it's not painful, but weird. Sometimes I get constipation which I never had before the surgery. It can be alleviated by fiber, however.

MA: All in all, did bariatric surgery give you what you were looking for?

R: Yes. I wish I had done it years ago.

MA: Is there something you wish you had known ahead of time?

R: Yes, how tough the adjustment period was. I didn't know how hard it would be to eat slowly and carefully and chew fully. These habits are hard to change even when the constant threat of choking and throwing up is in the back of my conscious mind. It's still hard and requires discipline. Cold foods and drink cause the banded esophagus to spasm if I'm not careful. That's hard to endure until the spasm goes away.

MA: What about the emotional impact of the surgery on you? The emotional impact of your weight loss and of other people's reactions?

R: What are these things: emotions? I'm a guy for heaven's sake! Emotions are what women have. Men have choices, needs, and habits. I have suffered from depression in my life but, for me, I've never equated depression with causing my overeating. I feel more natural now in my body instead of the fat cocoon I had been wearing. That said, my self-esteem has benefitted by fitting into smaller, trimmer clothes. But it makes me angry and frustrated from time to time that I'm not able to eat without fully concentrating. I really enjoy not being seen as morbidly obese by others. My family and friends are less worried about my health. They don't nag me or give me that silent, disapproving look about what I'm eating. And I don't feel guilty anymore about putting my family through worry.

MA: Do you still have cravings to overeat? How do you handle them?

R: Overeating is not an option. I am happy just to get down small portions. I never have cravings anymore, just occasional hunger which is satisfied by small portions. Since the surgery, I evaluate and consciously decide without compulsion when I'm hungry and what snack I want based solely on what I can get down easily. It's an amazing experience for me to take the time to consider what I would like to eat without mindlessly stuffing food down. I snack because it satisfies hunger—snacks are small and I can have anything I want because I know I won't gain weight. I eat ice cream, not because I crave it, but because it's easy going down and something I can truly enjoy eating without self-censoring.

MA: Anything I left out that could be relevant to understanding your decision?

R: After the surgery, I realized with amazement how many minutes of every day human social activity is centered around eating: shopping for food, deciding what to eat, cooking, eating, worrying about weight, cocktails, snacking, movies, parties. It's nice to be free of those concerns for most of the day. Leaves room for other thoughts and plans. Dinner with friends and family is less sociable because I now have to concentrate on eating carefully or I have to find a bathroom to throw up in. I warn people when I sit down to eat. I don't have lunch anymore with co-workers.

MA: Do you have any ongoing support?

R: My surgeon had a program of support groups, but I don't do support groups—Marlboro man kind of thing. I went on web sites which were helpful. One piece of advice I use: "Hiccups are your body's way of saying stop."

Robert has clearly achieved a successful outcome with his bariatric surgery which has made his life more healthy and enjoyable. Following the dramatic weight loss from the surgery, some people are strengthened in their resolve to cope better with overeating impulses. They are determined to sustain their new weight no matter what effort it takes.

Norma, like Robert, takes pride in her hard-won slenderness, works out regularly for the first time in her life, enjoys traveling for the first time, shopping for new clothes, and vows to do whatever she can to not return to her former size.

But some patients have psychological challenges afterward. Susan had a troubling reaction after her surgery—she began bingeing on alcohol and dropped out of her bariatric support group. And Joan became angry and depressed when she realized how much she would have to restrict her eating for the rest of her life. She felt robbed of being able to eat whatever she wanted when stressed out.

There are so many possible outcomes on the long-term effects of these surgeries that people contemplating bariatric surgery should consult with a mental health professional to evaluate if they have any emotional obstacles that could sabotage their success. These emotional roadblocks may include a history of depression or anxiety, physical or sexual abuse, drug or alcohol problems, or an isolated lifestyle with little social support.

Most of the overweight and obese patients I have treated have suffered from depression or anxiety and have used overeating to calm, soothe, and manage difficult feelings. Without learning new strategies to manage their feelings, weight loss surgery will not provide the cure for emotional eating. No amount of altering one's stomach size will address the psychological issues that can continue to fuel overeating. Philip, for example, underwent the stomach stapling procedure and, after initial weight loss, ate right through the staples back up to his former weight. Unable to cope with the onslaught of vulnerable feelings that arose with his thinner weight and smaller size, Philip, who had been beaten repeatedly as a child by his father, needed to restore his "protective" and hefty size to feel more emotionally secure.

Weight loss surgery stirs up controversy. The National Association to Advance Fat Acceptance (NAAFA) condemns gastrointestinal surgery for weight loss under any circumstance. They claim there is no conclusive evidence that this procedure increases longevity or improves overall health, although medical experience has indeed shown this surgery can reverse type 2 diabetes. NAAFA's studies have shown that hazards are downplayed on web sites and by surgeons, and there can be severe complications, including death. NAAFA advocates legislation to limit or control the weight-loss surgery industry and strongly recommends all patients be required to undergo psychological counseling prior to surgery.

The risks of weight loss surgery can include: excessive bleeding, infection, pulmonary embolism, blood clots, leaks in the gastrointestinal system, gallstones, dumping syndrome causing diarrhea, nausea or vomiting, and malnutrition such as iron deficiency.[31] Occasionally death does occur. One statistic claims the average is one in 350 people.[32]

A Comprehensive, Individualized Approach

Each organization dealing with obesity brings its own perspective and agenda to the table. Manufacturers of lap bands posit that the rise in obesity requires an increasing need for weight-loss surgery, and they now even recommend surgery for younger people as well. These companies are lobbying for medical insurance to provide larger reimbursements for weight-loss operations. An economic incentive is clearly present.

The Twelve Step program of Overeaters Anonymous, on the other hand, focuses on the addictive nature of overeating and claims many overweight and obese people are in denial about their compulsive eating and addiction to food. Breaking through denial is seen as the hallmark of recovery. Little acknowledgement is given to genetics as a cause for obesity.

National Association to Advance Fat Acceptance focuses on the influence of genetics and heredity in causing obesity, perhaps minimizing that, for some people, bingeing and overeating does contribute to weight gain.

Commercial weight-loss programs, also with a financial agenda, promote anxiety about how overweight is detrimental to one's health and the need to lose weight is paramount for success and happiness.

So, which group speaks the truth? In fact, each group has some validity to their position because every person's obesity is as unique as a fingerprint. No two obese people are created equal. Obesity and overweight are multi-determined conditions requiring an individualized approach for each person.

At the New York Center for Eating Disorders, we believe each person's overeating/overweight/obesity problem is different. Based on each person's individual needs, we blend a custom-tailored approach that includes psychotherapy, behavior modification to change negative thoughts and feelings about one's self, support groups, nutritional counseling, and/or medication. For some people, Overeaters Anonymous may be recommended; for others a nutritionist or one of the many commercial weight-loss programs. For a very select few, bariatric surgery may possibly be useful. A one-size approach to overeating/overweight/obesity does not fit all.

The Healing Role of Psychotherapy

One of the key ingredients to help people work through, resolve, and sustain their healing from compulsive overeating is psychotherapy.

Psychotherapy helps to improve a person's relationship with food, body image, and self-esteem. Psychotherapy teaches people how to develop the awareness to eat when physically hungry and not in response to emotional cravings. In therapy, people learn to identify and tolerate stressful emotions so they do not need to resort to eating to stuff down or divert themselves from these feelings. Therapy focuses on helping people develop better self-confidence by learning to identify and express feelings directly.

Psychotherapy can also play a role in helping someone break through their psychological resistance to exercise. I have worked with both men and women to untangle their inner, emotional conflicts to exercise. Wendy, for instance, had witnessed her father's death from a heart attack when she was a child and worried that exercise would place undue strain on her body and provoke her own heart attack. Discussing her concerns in therapy helped Wendy realize the distortion she harbored and how it was really her lack of activity that was unhealthy.

Another patient, Rose, had her jaw wired shut in a previous attempt to forcefully curtail her overeating. (This weight control method was sometimes used before the advent of bariatric surgery). The wires prevented her from overeating since she could basically only swallow a liquid diet. As we talked about why she decided to undergo jaw wiring, Rose explained how years of yo-yoing resulting in major weight loss followed by major weight gain led her to conclude she could not trust herself with food and needed to be restricted and even punished by this severe method.

Even with the wires in her mouth, Rose's urge to binge still tormented her. Rose recognized this desperate measure was doomed to fail in the long run because once the wires were removed, she had not really learned to eat healthfully or deal with the anxiety that led to her bingeing. In therapy, we helped Rose learn to manage her cravings with alternative behaviors, resolve some of her ongoing family problems, eat more healthfully, structure her meals, and introduce a regular exercise regime. We analyzed why she had always regained her lost weight in the past and worked to help her care for herself without jaw wiring. The ability to manage her feelings and food ultimately had to proceed from within, not from the external restriction of wires from without.

Victor, on the other hand, grew up with an athletic brother who became a professional tennis player. Knowing he could not compete with his brother's skill in sports made Victor retreat from doing any exercise. Therapy helped him challenge his all-or-nothing belief that either he had to be as good as his brother or he would not even try. Victor was able to adjust his competitive perspective and learn to get involved with exercise that was more suitable for him.

Victor's story highlights an important rule of thumb in working on an overweight or obesity problem: set small goals. New research indicates that losing even 10 percent of excess body weight can promote significant health benefits. Feeling overwhelmed about how much weight you have to lose will inevitably lead to despair and inertia. Instead, focus on losing this initial 10 percent, and then work to maintain it. Even if you never go beyond this point, you will be in a healthier place than yo-yoing up and down with a cycle of dramatic weight losses followed by weight gains.

Increasing exercise may be easier to put into practice than eating less because exercising does not necessarily provoke feelings of deprivation. Physical fitness improves your health much more than losing weight. People can be fit and fat which represents great progress over being unhealthy and fat.

Large men and women are often afraid or ashamed to exercise and may need to find creative ways to break through their reluctance, such as finding an exercise class for larger people. Many women report that taking a water aerobics class at a local Y is enjoyable and not threatening. Many overweight men report that choosing a gym that is low-key and not about macho guys parading around with huge biceps is more inviting and less intimidating.

Realistic Treatment Outcomes for Obesity and Overweight

No magic cure exists for obesity and overweight. But even if you come from a fat family with a genetic predisposition to be fat, you can still learn to separate your food from your feelings, unhook your eating from your emotions, and learn other coping strategies for stress.

You may never get to some "perfect" or "ideal" weight, but you do have other realistic options:

You can work to resolve emotional binge eating whether or not you lose weight.

You can stop the diet/binge cycle and become more attentive to inner signals of hunger and fullness. Diets do not work, and weight cycling is unhealthy.

You can become more fit and stronger through exercise. Fitness is the key to health, more than the number on the scale.

You can accept living in a larger body and refuse to be abusive to yourself or to accept mistreatment from others or society because of your size.

A new peace movement provides hope to obese and overweight people, the Health at Every Size movement. As the founder, Linda Bacon, states, "We're losing the war on obesity. Fighting fat has not made the fat go away. However, extensive 'collateral damage' has resulted: Food and body preoccupation, self-hatred, eating disorders, weight cycling, weight discrimination, poor health. . . . Few of us are at peace with our bodies, whether because we're fat or because we fear becoming fat. It's time to withdraw the troops. There is a compassionate alternative to an unjust war—Health at Every Size."

The HAES Manifesto states we can achieve peace and health through:

Accepting and respecting the diversity of body shapes and sizes in the world. That includes accepting *your* size!

Recognizing that health and well-being are multidimensional and that they include physical, social, spiritual, occupational, emotional, and intellectual aspects.

Promoting eating in a manner that balances individual nutritional needs, hunger, satiety, appetite, flexibility, and pleasure.

Promoting individually appropriate, enjoyable, life-enhancing physical activity, rather than exercise that is focused on the narrow goal of weight loss.[33]

As we discussed with anorexia, it can take a village to help overweight and obese people. I recommend putting together your own "personal team" of a doctor, nutritionist, individual therapist, personal trainer, and group therapy. Sometimes anti-anxiety or antidepressant medication can be helpful.

Whatever your weight, you do not need to be thin to start living and treating yourself well. Having a weight problem does not make you a bad person. The key is to leave no stone unturned to find a path that will help you live more healthfully and comfortably in your own body.

Whatever the method you chose to declare peace with your eating or weight problem, the significant ingredient is self-acceptance. If we are constantly waiting to get thin, we forget to live and enjoy our life. Life is not a dress rehearsal. As the soap opera title suggests, we only have "one life to live." And it is now. Let's commit to making it as satisfying as possible. Regardless of the number on the scale!

Night Eating Syndrome

"I'm so good and in control of my eating during the day," begins Nancy. "But then, after dinner and until I go to sleep, all hell breaks loose, and I can't stop eating. It's as if a vampire wakes up from inside me craving everything in sight."

I laugh and share with Nancy that I recently presented a professional paper which I entitled, "Binge Eating Disorder: Healing the Vampire Within." Many patients describe nighttime bingeing as akin to a voracious vampire stalking his next meal. Vampires and nighttime binge eaters have a lot in common: both are insatiable, they awake at night with ravenous hunger and ferociously launch into eating, indifferent to the consequences of their voracious rampages. Vampires and binge eaters both live to eat.

Symptoms of Night Eating Syndrome (NES)

You wake up in the morning not feeling hungry at all, you skip breakfast and perhaps drink lots of coffee to get yourself in gear.

You may skip lunch or just have something small. Nancy complained she was often too busy at work to even consider lunch and would just grab an apple or yogurt or another coffee. She wasn't sure whether or not she was hungry at this time of day.

You overeat at night because hunger from the day catches up with you. Restriction during the day invariably leads to compensating at night. Some people overeat at night because it is the first quiet, relaxing time in a busy day.

Margo described that only when her children and husband are asleep can she fully unwind, and nighttime bingeing is the treat she looks forward to all day. Some women may stay up at night to eat and to postpone going to bed so they can avoid unwanted sex. Other people report bingeing at night to energize themselves in order not to go to sleep. Reluctant for the day to end, wanting to squeeze in some extra personal time, they hope the food will keep them awake.

You eat at least one-third of your daily calorie intake after dinner.

You eat right up until the time you go to bed and then often have problems falling asleep. This may also be caused by excess intake of caffeine in coffee, tea, or soft drinks.

You wake up at night and raid the fridge, often worried that you won't be able to fall back to sleep without the comfort of the food.

You feel depressed or anxious or stressed which gives rise to the need to calm yourself by eating.

You wake up in the morning with a full stomach from nighttime eating, often with a food "hangover" and no desire to eat.

The vicious cycle starts all over again.

Night eating syndrome is different from binge eating and bulimia. Binge eaters and bulimics consume large amounts of food in one sitting. People with night-eating disorder may consume smaller snacks with high calorie content and wake up several times during the night to eat.

Sleeping difficulties are often linked to this syndrome. Nancy had chronic problems falling asleep and staying asleep and described excessive daytime sleepiness. Another patient, William, ate nothing during the day but began eating at 9 p.m. and continued for two hours. Two patients also reported sleepwalking in the middle of the night and raiding the refrigerator. They did not recall this activity until the following morning when they saw the telltale wrappers and crumbs on the kitchen counter.

Biological factors, such as hormones, play an important role in the development of NES which may be hereditary. Hormones can affect both eating and sleeping patterns. Psychological factors also contribute: in 75 percent of cases, depression and anxiety is associated with the onset of night eating. Women, with their fluctuating hormones and greater propensity to insomnia and depression, make up 60 percent of those with NES.

Plan of Action

Formulating concrete strategies to support your commitment to avoid night eating is key.

Increase your caloric intake during the day to prevent excess hunger at night. Restricting calories during the day will backfire at night, leading to overeating.

Re-establish regular meals and regular mealtimes with snacks as needed. Structure balanced meals with protein, carbohydrates, fruits and/or vegetables, and some fat. Many people do not eat dinner but graze all evening. This often contributes to NES. Kellie, who lived alone, would just have popcorn and a glass of wine for dinner in an attempt to lose weight. Not feeling satisfied, she would awake at night to eat again and then make herself throw up.

Eat breakfast whether or not you are hungry. Breakfast should include protein. People often object: "We never ate breakfast growing up in my family" or "I have no time in the morning" or "I hate breakfast." However, nobody is asking you to eat a four-course meal for breakfast. Just something. Breakfast revs up your metabolism and evens out your eating throughout the day.

Keep a food diary to monitor your eating patterns.

Establish a plan of exercise with at least 30 minutes of walking. However, intense exercise too close to bedtime may be over-stimulating and keep you awake.

Close down the television and computer an hour before sleep. The stimulation and the light from the screens can interfere with sleep; keep your bedroom dark. Some people find a white noise machine helpful as a sleep aid.

Before you go to sleep, set out foods that will not make you feel guilty if you wake up and eat them. Determine what food and how much will put you back to sleep.

Consult with your doctor or a psychiatrist about whether antidepressant medication or a temporary sleep medication might improve your mood and enhance the restorative quality of your sleep. Ask your doctor whether you need a sleep study to diagnose a possible sleep disorder, such as sleep apnea.

Consider a consultation with a psychotherapist to strategize your own unique plan of action.

Night eating syndrome did not begin overnight and will not go away overnight. Following a plan of action and getting help if you need it will put you on a path to health and wholeness again.

Men and Eating Disorders

Joseph called the New York Center for Eating Disorders in some distress, "I think I have an eating disorder and would like to make an appointment. I bet I'm the first man who's ever called you about an eating problem."

"Actually," I responded, "many men have eating problems. They're just not as brave as you to pick up the phone and get some help."

Joseph expresses a common misconception—that eating disorders are problems of girls and women, not men. In truth, more women than men do have anorexia, bulimia, or binge eating disorders, but men are not exempt from these struggles. Experts estimate that 10 to 15 percent of people with eating disorders are male, but this figure may be low. Many men suffer in silence and feel too ashamed to bring this issue to their doctor or a therapist. Men may also be under-represented in the statistics of eating disorders because they can hide their eating problems better than women. An overweight man with a binge eating disorder is less the object of ridicule than an overweight woman. Our society is more tolerant and forgiving of extra pounds on men, while women are held to a stricter standard. Also, men who are obsessed with working out and building muscle may be admired as strong, macho guys, which can camouflage their suffering and anxiety about their body image or hide an eating disorder.

During his therapy consultation, Joseph, a 24-year-old, described his upset over his girlfriend, Sherry, leaving him for another man. Joseph felt rejected and concluded that if he were thinner, he would be more handsome, and Sherry would have stayed with him. He had embarked on a strict dieting regime to make himself feel more attractive and boost his self-esteem. But his under-eating backfired. He found himself bingeing and then making himself throw up.

Joseph revealed he had always felt clumsy as a boy, was only half-heartedly picked for team sports, and felt inadequate compared to his father who had played varsity football many years ago. Joseph considered his father more masculine than himself. Joseph's story highlights some particular dynamics that may trigger male eating disorders:

Low self-esteem and anxieties about one's masculinity.
Unfavorably comparing oneself to other men, be it a brother, a father, or peers.
Feeling inadequate in competing with other men in activities such as sports or dating.

Other factors that increase male vulnerability toward developing body dissatisfaction and eating disorders include a man who:

Was fat or overweight as a child. To be a fat boy is to be thought a sissy, *whether or not the boy is gay.*

May have looked effeminate.

Was bullied or teased by family or peers.

Identified and modeled himself after his mother's or sister's dieting preoccupations.

Had an obese father.

Participates in a sport that requires thinness or weight control—running, bodybuilding, wrestling.

Has a job or profession that requires thinness—male models, actors.

Has anxieties about his sexuality. Some men may have a sexual identity conflict. To them, fat = female and, therefore, any fat on their bodies will reveal to the world their feminine self. Being fat can feel like a threat because it means to be round and womanly, like mother.

Is homosexual. Gay culture is known to highly value a thin, muscular physique.

Has a history of physical or sexual abuse. This can fracture the ability to trust and love others and trust and love one's self. Bingeing, purging, or starving can become a substitute "intimate" relationship.

Our media is replete with images depicting what a "real man" should look like: buff, with buns of steel and six-pack abs. Muscular sports figures and handsome actors, often with steroid-enhanced bodies, dominate the male imagination. These unattainable, airbrushed, perfect male bodies can induce the same kind of insecurities that women have suffered with for so long. Men's health magazines reflect (or provoke) male anxieties with articles like, "Sex: Seduce Her with Style," "Double Your Sexual Stamina," "Are You A Lousy Kisser?," "15 Minutes to Get Ripped," "Build an Immortal Body."[34]

Even young boys are getting the macho body image message early. Action figures for young boys, such as G.I. Joe, have progressively increased their muscular, bulging physique, sending the message to boys that the appearance of brute strength is everything and only bigger is better. This is parallel to how the Barbie doll, with her exaggerated measurements, has influenced young girls' perceptions of how a sexy woman should look.[35]

However, a curious cultural contradiction is now afoot. On one hand, men are admired for working out and becoming brawny while, at the same time, an article in *Psychology Today* titled "Manorexic Mannequins" describes how ultra-thin males are now coming into vogue. A famed British mannequin maker debuts the latest male form—the 'Homme Nouveau,' feminized and not so hearty . . . Perfect for the trendiest, string beaniest clothing."[36]

The changes of male mannequin shapes since the 1960s are significant:[37]

The Classic	1967	42 inch chest	33 inch waist
The Muscleman	1983	41 chest	31 waist
The Swimmer	1994	38 chest	28 waist
Homme Nouveau	2010	35 chest	27 waist

These shifting images promote an increase in male body image dissatisfaction, giving rise to a new diagnostic category, "male body dysmorphia." MBD refers to the distortion in how men perceive their bodies. While the anorexic girl persists in feeling fat despite being emaciated, the man with body dysmorphia represents the opposite side of the coin: He views himself as inferior, undeveloped, or scrawny *even though he may be well-built and strong.* No matter how much he works out, his feelings of smallness and inadequacy still persist. This is a *psychological* distortion with an overlay of cultural messages dictating how "real" men should look.

Men who are eager to increase their muscle strength have turned to steroids in record numbers. Use of anabolic steroids, synthetic forms of the hormone testosterone, is on the rise. (Ironically, side effects include female-like breast development and lowered testosterone levels as well as spikes of aggressive behavior referred to as 'roid rage). Many men's magazines and online web sites provide an array of advertisements to purchase the muscle-building supplements, pituitary growth hormones, and black market steroids. "Steroidology" is the underground world of bodybuilders, who trade tips on fat-burning products and muscle enhancers with names as enticing as "Universal Animal Rage," "Muscle Milk," "Fountain of Youth," "Anabolic Addiction Mass Addiction Amplified," and "Horny Goat Weed." Other sites and ads target male insecurities around hair loss and penis size (referred to as "the penis enlargement industry").[38]

Men are more willing than ever to have "work done." According to the American Society for Aesthetic Plastic Surgery, procedures for men are up more than 300 percent since 1997. Some men, who are driven to look brawny with bulging chests and slender waists, resort to liposuction. Other men seek saline implants to enhance their chests' pectoral muscles and also may have six saline packets inserted to define the "six-pack" ripped abdomen muscles. Men increasingly believe plastic surgery may give them an edge in the competitive, youth-oriented corporate world.

Unlike women celebrities, few famous men have come forward to discuss their eating disorder struggles. One exception is actor Dennis Quaid who has talked about his battle with "manorexia," for which he sought treatment. Quaid said his problem started when he lost 40 pounds to play Doc Holliday in the 1994 movie *Wyatt Earp*. Actor Billy Bob Thornton revealed he, too, has battled anorexia, at one point losing 59 pounds, and singer Elton John admitted he suffered from bulimia. Former male model Ron Saxen describes his ordeal with binge eating and abuse history in one of the few eating disorder books written from a male perspective.[39]

Men, Sexuality, and Eating Disorders

Our culture places undue stress and anxiety on young men to be hyper-sexual. Increasingly, the image of the ideal man is a powerful stud, Don Juan, ladies' man, macho man, smooth operator, he-man, virile, a jock, a guy with a "big package." Common exhortations include "love 'em and leave 'em" or "find 'em, feel 'em, fuck 'em, forget 'em." Adolescent boys may feel pressure and conflict about living up to this inflated masculine persona.

Some may retreat from the pressure to be sexual by reverting to anorexia, bulimia, or binge eating disorder (or alcohol and drugs). Kenneth came to treatment for anorexia. Although *many* factors figured into his developing an eating disorder, he admitted to feeling shocked and inhibited starting at age 14 when his father bragged about having slept with over 500 women. Fearful he could never compete with such an exalted number of lovers, Kenneth became depressed and retreated to the safety of social isolation and severe food restriction; he lost his appetite for food and for sex. His eating disorder kept him in a state of sexual "hibernation," because self-starvation reduces a man's testosterone level and sex drive.

Kenneth's therapy helped him recognize and work through the lifelong competition his father had thrust on him in many arenas. And we discussed how, when it came to sex, savoring the experience of making love could be much more enjoyable than obsessing about scratching another notch on the bedpost of how many women he had conquered! Kenneth began humming the Frank Sinatra song, "I Did It My Way" as a reminder that *his* pleasure and experiences were what were truly meaningful.

Sexual abuse, with its residue of suppressed rage and feeling like damaged goods, can also trigger an eating disorder. The Center for Disease Control and Prevention reported that one in 71 men admitted they had been raped, with one-quarter assaulted before they were age ten, usually by someone they know. Other estimates have run even higher. The Department of Justice reports one in 33 men has been sexually abused. "Like women, men who are raped feel violated and ashamed and may become severely depressed. . . . They are at increased risk for substance abuse, problems with interpersonal relationships, physical impairments, insomnia . . . and also face a challenge to their sense of masculinity."[40] And I would add, they are also at increased risk for eating disorders.

Paul was sexually abused by his sister's husband. James began molesting Paul when he was 11 years old, and, at age 13, Paul developed bulimia. Paul was filled with self-disgust at what he believed was his fat and ugly body and would accuse himself unmercifully for being a bad person when he binged and threw up and used laxatives. Like so many people who suffer from emotional eating, Paul transformed an intensely horrific sexual abuse experience by his brother-in-law into the familiar pain about how fat he was. Familiar pain is more endurable than anguish over which we have no control.

Paul eventually confided his ordeal to his mother, "My mother told me that since the experience (she called it experience, not abuse!) had stopped last year when I turned 15, there was no point in confronting James now and ruining my sister's marriage. 'Let bygones be bygones,' she said. 'Maybe you're exaggerating. Anyway, you're fine now. I can't believe he meant anything bad.' It had taken me so much courage to finally tell her, and now she says the family will get ruined if I tell the truth out loud and that it will be my fault. I'm devastated she's choosing to protect James and my sister over me." His mother's response made the experience even more traumatic—a double betrayal.

In his therapy, Paul "threw up" massive amounts of rage and pain and purged himself with words, not food. Paul came to feel justified in his rage and felt sorrow for himself for being victimized. His capacity to cry and grieve the betrayal by both his brother-in-law and his mother was crucial to his recovery. By going through the process of uncovering the emotions beneath the surface of his bulimia, he eventually healed his eating problem, although the scars of betrayal and mistrust still remain.

Paul also became a member of MaleSurvivor.Org, a group committed to healing and preventing the sexual victimization of men and boys. He began joining their forums and attending conferences. MaleSurvivor.Org provided a missing piece in Paul's recovery—the opportunity to interact, share, and recover with other men who had suffered the effects of abuse.[41]

Homosexuality and Eating Disorders

The documentary film, *Do I Look Fat: Gay Men, Body Image and Eating Disorders,* presents a series of interviews with homosexual men. The film uncovered a remarkable statistic: "While just 5 percent of men are thought to be gay, that 5 percent represents up to 40 percent of men with eating disorders . . . In up to 50 percent of male patients, conflicts over gender identity precipitated the development of an eating disorder."[42]

While many men recognize and embrace their homosexuality without apology, others are in conflict regarding:

Anguish over being different, unsure, or uncertain about their gender identity.

Anxious about coming out and declaring oneself.

Fear of reactions from family, peers, and colleagues.

Although a man may declare he is gay, this does not necessarily mean he is fully self-accepting. Society's homophobia can become internalized and cause the boy or man turmoil over his sexual identity.

As one man in the documentary revealed, "My self-esteem about my sexual orientation made me turn to food. Food was a relief; it made my head and emotions blank."

A sampling of other comments from the men in the film:

"Which is worse—to be fat or a fag?"

"I didn't know how I felt about being gay, so I chose anorexia."

"There is so much fat phobia in the gay community. But you can't be too thin either or people will think you have AIDS."

"I have to be punished [with an eating disorder] because I didn't walk or talk like a man and my father disapproved of me."

"I was afraid of contact with women so I tried to eat away the anxiety. I ate myself into a coma."

"We oppress ourselves when there is no one left to oppress us.

"Not eating is a form of oppression—a way to disappear because getting [gay male] attention is too painful."

Treating Male Eating Disorders

The first medical report of a man with an eating disorder was recorded in 1694 by a London physician, Dr. Richard Morton. He described a male anorexic patient as suffering from "Nervous Consumption" caused by "Sadness and Anxious Cares." He prescribed "a resting cure of horseback riding and abstention from studies." Unfortunately, contemporary treatment approaches don't much subscribe to horseback riding or neglecting one's school work or job in order to get better!

A more contemporary treatment includes the case of Dave, a successful businessman with a family of five young children. Although he had been athletic as a younger man, the demands of his business, traveling for work, and supporting his family eroded his opportunity to exercise. Dave described coming home from work and raiding the refrigerator before and after dinner. No matter how much food his wife Meryl prepared, Dave was not content unless he was stuffing himself throughout the evening. He was gaining weight, and his wife urged him to get help.

In therapy, Dave came to see that bingeing was his method to de-stress, to shift gears after an intense work day. Overeating was his reward to himself for his grueling schedule, but it was beginning to take its toll on his health and appearance. Dave initially felt selfish to admit he needed some private time for himself, given that Meryl took care of the house and their five children all day. But, much to his surprise, Meryl supported his efforts to break the binge cycle by going to therapy, joining a gym, and working out with a trainer.

We explored why Dave always put himself at the bottom of the list of people to be taken care of. We discovered this was related to his helping to support his original family from an early age because of his father's ill health. Recognizing this pattern from his youth illuminated Dave's need to change his behavior with his present-day family. He came to see the importance of his own need for self-care. "I always assumed that to be a man meant being the family provider and bread-winner who sucked it all up without complaint. Therapy helped me realize that the reason my father died young was that he never gave himself a break, never ate well or exercised, just worked, worked, worked. My wish to 'man up' to all my responsibilities is going to lead to one 'man down'—me, six feet under! I vow to do everything in my power not to leave Meryl a widow or my children without a dad. I'm off to the gym now! I feel more liberated and no longer such a slave to my job or overeating."

Eating disorder therapy for men, as well as for women, involves creating a comprehensive treatment plan based on the unique needs of each person. This involves giving up restrictive, depriving dieting as well as designing behavioral strategies to change unwanted eating patterns. Psychotherapy also involves bringing into awareness those emotional issues that block a man from unfolding into an integrated and contented person.

Men with eating problems can be helped. Sometimes it takes some extra courage to reach out for that help.[43]

Pregnancy and Eating Disorders

"Look how fat I've gotten," Valerie points with dismay at her eight-month pregnant belly.

"If Angelina Jolie can get back in shape right after having twins, why can't I?" demands Elaine.[44]

"My husband and I are trying to get pregnant, but it's just not happening. Do you think it has to do with my bulimia?" worries Carla.

For most women, a planned pregnancy is an exciting event as they watch their bellies grow to accommodate their new baby. That doesn't mean it is all smooth sailing physically or emotionally, but the overwhelming feeling is, "This is awesome!"

But for women with eating disorders, pregnancy is a time when body image concerns intensify. A woman may feel powerless over her growing body and her increased appetite and weight. She may also fear that her pregnancy means she is now going to be fat forever. These fears and emotional discomfort have the potential to lead her back to bingeing, purging, or restricting.

Certain at-risk women may also develop "pregorexia," a term used to describe pregnant women so obsessed with keeping their weight in check that they diet and exercise excessively, potentially endangering their unborn babies. These women focus on "starving for two."[45]

Fertility

A woman's history of anorexia, bulimia, or compulsive overeating should not necessarily prevent her from becoming pregnant. Leslie gave birth to two children, despite a lifelong history of bulimia. Stephanie is now pregnant with her third child, despite long-term anorexia, food restriction, and irregular menstrual periods since her teenage years.

However, an eating disorder can often disrupt the delicate balance of hormones that control ovulation, menstruation, and conception. Without sufficient body fat, a woman ceases to get her period and, therefore, may not get pregnant. At least half the women with anorexia, bulimia, or binge eating disorder may suffer from irregular periods. Women with a body mass index lower than 18.5 have an increased risk of miscarriage.

Some women are reluctant to openly discuss their eating problems due to shame or fear they may have impaired their fertility. But it is essential, before undergoing arduous and expensive fertility treatments, that a woman discuss any past or present eating problems with her doctor. Sometimes treatment for an eating disorder can be the key step to enhance fertility. Postponing pregnancy until you have improved your eating disorder may also be an option to consider.

Pregnancy

Your eating disorder is *not* your fault. It is a blend of heredity, biology, psychology, habits, social pressure, and spiritual illness. But getting help *is* your responsibility.

Several binge eaters in my practice reported with surprise and delight that their overeating lessened or even resolved when they were pregnant. The tenderness and loving anticipation for their growing baby allowed them to feed themselves with increased attentiveness to healthy eating. Vicki related, "It's one thing to hurt myself with bingeing, but it's unacceptable I should hurt my innocent baby."

The International Journal of Eating Disorders published a research study that corroborates what I have found to be true.[46] The study shows pregnancy had a beneficial impact on anorexia and bulimia symptoms. Lasting psychological benefit, however, often requires further treatment to support the progress made during pregnancy.

"Be your own good mother," I advised Vicki after she gave birth. "You ate well for your baby; now let's help you do it for yourself. Let's apply what you did while pregnant to your very own self as if there is a little Vicki living inside of you who needs you to care and feed her with love."

Women who conceive while suffering from anorexia or bulimia can jeopardize both their own health and the health of the fetus. Anorexia, purging, and laxative or diuretic abuse can seriously deplete the pregnant mom's nutritional reserves, and she may experience the exhaustion and depression that accompanies malnourishment. Also, the fetus may be robbed of sufficient nutrients as it tries to take nourishment from a depleted mother.

Eating disorders affect pregnancy with these possible complications:

Premature labor
Low birth weight
Stillbirth or fetal death
Increased risk of caesarean birth
Delayed fetal growth
Respiratory problems
Gestational diabetes
Complications during labor
Depression
Miscarriage
Preeclampsia (high blood pressure)

Guidelines for Pregnancy and Eating Disorders
Before getting pregnant:

A woman with an active eating disorder can improve her chances of having a healthy baby. You should work toward achieving and maintaining a healthy weight with support from your doctor, nutritionist, and/or therapist. Your eating does not have to be perfect, just better. Progress, not perfection. It is healthier to keep your weight stable, even if it is higher than you would prefer, rather than yo-yoing up and down. Prenatal vitamins can help restore the body's level of vitamins, minerals, and calcium.

Avoid purging to the best of your ability. A bulimic patient, Lucy, came up with her personal strategy, "the delay tactic." Unsure she could be free of bulimia for the rest of her life, Lucy decided that once her baby was born she could then go back to bulimia if she needed to. By giving herself permission to return to bulimia in the future, she helped sustain her resolve while pregnant. Her resolution while pregnant was, "Do not make yourself throw up, no matter what. If I'm really honest, I know the difference between morning sickness and purging." After Chloe's birth, she shifted to, "I'll throw up tomorrow if I want." This postponement strategy worked well for her because she did not want anyone, including herself, to tell her she could never be bulimic again.

During pregnancy:

Strive for a healthy weight gain. Most doctors recommend about 25 to 35 pounds, but each individual may have a different requirement.

Discuss your eating disorder with your healthcare professional. For the sake of the baby, this is not a time for secrecy. Ask for suggestions about how much exercise is optimal and what the limitations may be.

If you are an overweight binge eater, you may have a higher risk of preeclampsia (high blood pressure) and gestational diabetes and may need to be monitored more frequently.

Many studies have suggested "that what, and how much, a mother eats during pregnancy can 'program' a child's organ systems before birth and set the stage for metabolic or hormonal changes that may result in disease many years later. The major damage is caused by maternal undernutrition. . . . Small size, meaning under 5.5 pounds, can result in a 35 percent higher rate of coronary deaths in later life and a six-fold increase in the risk of diabetes or impaired glucose metabolism."

On the other hand, "excessive weight gain in pregnancy can result in bigger-than-average babies who are prenatally programmed to become overweight children—who, in turn, are more likely to develop diabetes, heart disease and cancer later in life."[47]

After pregnancy:

Develop a healthy food plan that is realistic. All women need patience and time to deal with postpartum weight gain. Be compassionate with yourself. You just delivered a new little being into the world!

If you are breastfeeding, be sure to get adequate nutrition. Otherwise you will pass along any vitamin deficiencies to the baby.

Ask for the support you need from your doctor, therapist, and/or nutritionist.

Recognize the symptoms of postpartum depression. This is not uncommon in women with eating disorders. Do not suffer in silence. Ask for help. Seek treatment. You are not alone.

Becoming a new mother—whether it's your first child or your seventh—is stressful and exhausting. Often a new mom forgets to nurture herself. If you have struggled with an eating disorder, remember that factoring yourself into the equation of self-care is especially crucial so you do not get depleted which leads to emotional eating. Get as much sleep as possible, take a break from the baby from time to time, don't lose touch with your partner, and remember, the investment is worth it: Your baby *will* grow up, you *will* eventually sleep, and you *will* reclaim ownership of your body once again!

Older Women, Body Image, and Eating Disorders

> I'm selfish, impatient and a little insecure. I make mistakes, I
> am out of control and at times hard to handle. But if you can't
> handle me at my worst, then you sure as hell don't deserve me
> at my best.
>
> —Marilyn Monroe

I am outdoors at a Miami spa, finishing up the morning water aerobics class. I am sweaty and disheveled in the 90-degree heat, while the woman next to me in the pool looks like she just came from a beauty makeover session. Her eye makeup and mascara are not dripping, her lipstick is coral perfection, and her cheek blush is as intact as when we started the class an hour ago in the Florida sun.

"Your makeup looks gorgeous," I turn to her with curiosity.

"I know," she laughs, "my makeup is permanently tattooed on!"

I'm astonished. I've never heard of this. She is friendly and I come closer to peer at her face.

Gwen confides, "I had the tattooing done last year. I figured who wouldn't want to wake up every day looking perfect and all put together?"

I think about her question for a while. There is something tempting about hopping out of bed every morning looking radiant with coral lip color (goes with any outfit!) and coral blush and moon pearl eye shadow to enhance the color of your eyes. And you would never have to fish in your pocketbook ever again for that elusive lipstick. Tempting . . .

But would I feel pressure to live up to a constantly flawless face? I begin to realize I really do want the expression on my face to match my inner mood. If I'm in a bad mood, well, maybe I want everyone to know it. If I have the flu, how could I get my husband to bring me chicken soup in bed if I look fresh as a daisy? I decide a frozen face and perfect makeup is not for me. But it was fun fantasizing for awhile.

Body image preoccupation and eating disorders are not just the domain of teenage girls. Middle-aged and older women worry about their weight, their size, and what they eat. Nowadays, middle-aged women may seek out liposuction, Botox, and plastic surgery in an anxious attempt to "restore" themselves to a younger, firmer self.

Given that the average life expectancy for a woman in the United States is 78 years, a woman reaches midlife around 39. That's a lot of years left to work on making peace with one's body growing older!

Psychoanalyst and author Judith Viorst, speaks in *Necessary Losses,* of the necessity of accepting the loss of one's own younger self, "the self that thought it would be unwrinkled, invulnerable and immortal." In her book, *How Did I Get to Be 40 and Other Atrocities,* Viorst captures the rue and regret many women feel about the unrelenting passage of time: While I was thinking I was just a girl / My future turned into my past.[48]

An article in *Oprah* magazine asks: "What Scares Women About Getting Older? *Everything!*" And a recent glance through several women's magazines reveals advertisements for Youth Dew, Damage Remedy, anti-wrinkle firming lotion, Deception (to erase your wrinkles), anti-aging serum, elasticity boost, intensive rebuilding cream, reshaping and lifting crème, age reversal technology, and perfectionist correcting serum.

And what about these names? Are they dinosaurs recently unearthed by archaeologists? Newly discovered viruses? Lost tribes of the Amazon?

Pitera, pre-tocopheryl, retinaldehyde, polyolprepolymers, C8 peptides, zeatin, kinetin, chitosan, silica silylate, fullerene, decapeptide-12, ascorbyl tetraisopalmitate, acyl-glutathione, Anogeissus, idebenone, poly-L-lactic acid, neurosensine, ascorbyl tetraisopalmitate, Melaplex complex, polidocanol

No! These are ingredients for "age-defying" facial products.[49]

Humor: The Antidote to the Anxiety of Aging

Middle age is when your age starts to show around your middle.
—Bob Hope

Have humor! Some women, fortunately, learn to deal with their chang-ing bodies with humor rather than self-loathing, knowing that all of us have to go through the journey of getting older. Anna Magnani, the voluptuous Italian actress, laughingly said about the bags under her eyes: "A whole lot of good living went into making this face of mine!"

Gypsy Rose Lee affirmed: "I have everything I had 20 years ago, only it's all a little bit lower."

Bette Davis declared: "Old age is no place for sissies."

And Dolly Parton jokes, "I'm not offended by all the dumb blonde jokes because I know I'm not dumb—and I also know I'm not blonde!"

At age 20 I studied in Spain for my college junior year abroad. By 1998, I am 50 years old, and my husband and I have decided to take a vacation to Sevilla. We plan to meet up with my old Spanish boyfriend, Antonio, whom I dated when we were studying at the Universidad de Sevilla. We will have dinner and I will meet his wife Teresa for the first time. It has been 30 years since I've seen Antonio.

"I really hope I'm prettier than Teresa!" I think to myself.

I cannot believe that this unbidden thought pops into my head! I cannot believe that I—a feminist, a therapist, a happily married wom-an, and very well psychoanalyzed—should have such an immature reaction to our meeting. I've reduced this whole reunion into anxiety about whether or not I'm prettier than Teresa! I sheepishly confide this to my husband. Michael responds laughingly, "Well, I was secretly hoping that I'm stronger than Antonio. That way I can beat him up if I see he still loves you!" We laugh uproariously.

As I speak on the phone with Antonio to make our dinner plans, he warns me in Spanish, "Well, I now have a lot less hair than I did 30 years ago when you knew me." I think to myself, "I remember you were bemoaning your balding head even back when we were in our 20s." This is hilarious. Here we are—three middle-aged folks— reverting at a moment's notice to the teenage body preoccupations, comparisons, and competitions of three decades ago. And who knows what Teresa is thinking!

A few older actresses and models have managed to retain their youthful appearance. An article in *The New York Post* declares: "Here's Lauren Hutton at the age of 62—looking hotter than most models do at 26. The super-sexy star . . . strikes a blow for older women everywhere."

But for most of us, it's hard to look as glamorous as Lauren Hutton—even when we're younger! And actor Kathleen Turner empathizes. At age 58, she lashed out at American movie directors who only hire actresses below a certain age. "I'm going to Italy. I think they respect women of my age more. In Europe, they see more the entire body of work, as opposed to simply how you look today. . . . . Our culture is very youth-oriented, and I don't really understand why because it's not very interesting. I like to be comfortable in my body. I don't want to think about every bite of food I put in my mouth to maintain a certain weight. I don't want to get all the surgery."

The actor Charlotte Rampling, at age 66, also believes older actresses should proudly face their age. "The camera can be unforgiving, much more so than we see ourselves. But it's quite moving to see a woman who was once young and beautiful—you see time turning."

At age 68, Lauren Hutton affirmed, "Wrinkles are our medals of the passage of life."

Diane Keaton, at age 66, declared herself against plastic surgery as a matter of integrity, "I want to express my age and be authentic."

Actress Maggie Smith, at age 77, "Puts to rest the idea that women should hold tight to a particular age, a particular look, rather than giving their faces permission to move through the life cycle."[50]

Jane Fonda, at 74, and Sally Field, at 64, swore off any more nips and tucks. As Fonda stated in *Glamour* in 2007, "I realized [when she was going to be 70], I have chosen not to have any more plastic surgery. Sally and I have kind of made a pact about that. It's really hard, especially when you're a public person. But I want to give a face to aging." (This is a healthy evolution from Fonda's once bulimic self, she has made an "about-face" from her previous cosmetic surgeries and breast implants; no pun intended!)[51]

Fonda asserts: "I'm trying to organize my friends and women in my profession to say no to the duck lips and to let the wrinkles happen naturally. I've just traveled through Sweden and Finland looking at faces that were real. They had their life experiences on them as opposed to in Hollywood where everybody is starting to look alike."

But despite Fonda's efforts to help older women feel better about themselves, Joanne Woodward complained that, until he died, actor husband Paul Newman got handsomer every year, while she just got older.

And on her 40th birthday, Grace Kelly lamented that although 40 was a terrific age for a man, it was torture for a woman because it was the beginning of the end.

Ingrid Bergman said: "When you look at yourself in the mirror every morning . . . you don't realize you're aging. But then you find a friend who was young with you and the friend isn't young anymore, then all of a sudden you remember you too aren't young anymore."

Cher said: "In my job becoming old and becoming extinct are one and the same thing."

During a visit to the United States in 2005, shortly after marrying England's Prince Charles, Camilla Parker Bowles was described in the *New York Post* and *Daily News* as a "frump" and "dowdy and past her prime." Cartoons showed her as an aging horse. Her real sin?

Being a middle-aged woman in her late 50s trying to look glamorous.

Comparing Princess Diana to Camilla, Andrea Peyser of the *New York Post* unleashed this catty remark: "Buckingham Palace has traded in its resident high drama, depression and bulimia [of Princess Diana] for laugh lines, liver spots and middle-age spread. Cutting and suicide attempts are out, face-lifts and cosmetic dentistry in."

Quentin Letts of the *Wall Street Journal* had a kinder impression of this older woman: "The first stop of Prince Charles and Camilla Parker Bowles was a party in Manhattan. On the guest list that evening: middle-aged males and their trophy women. Some of the older broads, dolled up like vintage Barbies, had undergone near-industrial levels of plastic surgery. Few seemed convincingly happy. Camilla is a mature, warm woman, well lived-in like a country club armchair. She dresses sensibly without upstaging others. . . . Yes, she has laughter lines. Sure, she'll never make a living as a *Vogue* mannequin. But is this lady not a model for our age? Isn't she more truly admirable? Give the old girl a chance, America."[52]

Even William Shakespeare described the beleaguered aging female in a Sonnet:

> *When forty winters shall besiege thy brow*
> *And dig deep trenches in thy beauty's field,*
> *Thy youth's proud livery, so gazed on now,*
> *Will be a tattered weed of small worth held.*

In other words, Shakespeare proclaims, after age 40 a woman ain't so hot!

However, Shakespeare did have to admit that Cleopatra would always be beautiful despite her years: "Age cannot wither her, nor custom stale her infinite variety."

As Maureen Dowd, *New York Times* columnist, puts it: "Men can look good in many different ways, whereas women are expected to endlessly replicate themselves at twenty-five, à la Goldie Hawn and Heather Locklear, until they look like frozen reproductions of themselves. Our culture is obsessed with freezing the clock—and the face—with lifestyle drugs and medical treatments . . . I worry that women are heading toward one face. Sometimes in affluent settings, you see a bunch of eerily similar women with oddly off-track features—Botox-smoothed, Formica foreheads, collagen-protruding lips, surgically narrowed noses, taut jaws—who look like sisters from another planet."[53]

Plastic surgery does, indeed, scramble individuality.

When we reflect on the glamorous women of the past, each had her own iconic signature look and reveled in her unique beauty and distinctive style. How different Sophia Loren was from Audrey Hepburn, or Elizabeth Taylor from Bette Davis, or Katherine Hepburn from Marilyn Monroe. It is astonishing to realize that the actors we admire today as younger women are also aging, just like the rest of us. None of us is exempt!

In 2012, at the age of 90, Iris Apfel, style icon and textile magnate, became the inspiration for a new line of cosmetics, making her the oldest woman to personally represent a line of beauty products. Her gloriously aged face looked forthrightly, unapologetically from the publicity photo of the cosmetics store display.

As an anonymous writer, pondering how short life really is, once declared, "Do not regret growing older. It is a privilege denied to many."

Eating Disorders and Older Women

Robyn called the New York Center for Eating Disorders with some anxiety, "I am a 58-year-old woman with bulimia. I know this is supposed to be a problem of high school girls. Is it too late for me to get help?"

It is true that eating disorders usually affect younger women during the teenage years or early 20s. But these disorders can also begin later in life, affecting women in their 30s, 40s, 50s, and older. No age is immune from developing an eating disorder.

Adulthood is filled with challenges, some dramatic, some subtle. These changes can test our identity and stress our coping abilities. Many adult women inevitably have to confront the empty nest when their children leave home. Sometimes this causes a couple's identity crisis as a new kind of relationship between husband and wife needs to evolve. In addition, a woman may have other issues—menopause, retirement, caregiving for older parents, and possible illness. When forced to cope with such uncomfortable transitions/emotional disruptions, people often begin to obsess about their bodies and translate complicated feelings into the language of fat.

Robyn became bulimic as a teenager and never resolved it, despite the success of a professional career, marriage, and motherhood. It was her private, shameful secret. With the death of her parents, her three grown children leaving home, and her husband struggling with setbacks in his business, Robyn's bulimia escalated, and she came for help for the first time.

In Robyn's case, we came to understand that she resorted to bingeing, purging, and preoccupation with weight as a way to avoid confronting her sad and insecure reactions to these losses.

The eating disorders of older women usually occur with one of three possibilities:

A woman develops an eating disorder as a teenager, never resolves it, and it persists through various stages of her life.

Gail, a 60-year-old woman, was very close to her only son, Jerry. When Jerry and his wife had their first child, the couple became absorbed with the baby. Gail felt left out and jealous of her son's relationship with the baby. When Jerry and his family moved out of state, Gail's jealousy intensified. She felt guilty and ashamed of her feelings. She began to binge.

In her therapy, we discovered that jealousy had also been an issue for Gail as a teenager. When she did not feel as popular as the other girls in high school and at different junctures in her adult life, she would binge as a way to comfort herself and to discharge angry feelings. Making this connection between her teenage struggles and current emotions helped Gail explore her life-long vulnerability to feeling unimportant. She faced her past history of feeling left out and neglected. Once she identified these emotions and worked through her guilt, she no longer needed to detour her anger through binge eating. Gail also became less ashamed about communicating with her son the genuine need for the family connection she was yearning for.

A woman develops an eating disorder as a teenager, succeeds in resolving it for a period of time, but relapses as an older woman.

Sara discovered that her husband was having an affair. Unable to directly face her anger and grief, Sara relapsed to anorexia, which she had suffered from periodically at various challenging times in her life, starting at age 14 when her parents divorced. Given that Sara was financially dependent on her husband, she was particularly scared to voice the full brunt of her fury and hurt. Instead, she diverted her rage into a silent protest by not eating. The language of pain comes in many dialects. Sara recruited her body to express what she could not say in words. She went on a hunger strike.

Concern for his wife's health and a sincere wish to stay in the marriage prompted Todd to agree to couple's counseling. Together they began to sort out what had derailed their marriage and how to repair it. Sara felt nurtured by her husband's interest in saving their relationship. As she began to communicate her pain directly, she no longer had to resort to starving herself as a way of silently venting her anger and despair.

A woman begins suffering from an eating disorder or body image dissatisfaction for the first time as an adult.

Danya was 41 when she accidentally became pregnant with her sixth child. She had been looking forward to more time for herself now that her children were older, and she was distressed about the arrival of the new baby and "getting fat all over again." As a religious woman, ending the pregnancy was not an option. Danya began suffering from bulimia for the first time in her life in an attempt to purge her guilt about her "bad" feelings, which she considered "sinful and selfish." Through her therapy, Danya came to understand her regret over this unplanned pregnancy was a natural reaction for someone who thought her days of mothering an infant were over. She felt understood and validated in her therapy and entitled to her feelings of dismay. Danya discussed this ambivalence with her husband, who admitted to similar feelings as well. Sharing their reactions with each other increased their closeness and helped them become more eager about the new addition to their family.

Although Gail, Sara, and Danya each developed an eating disorder at different phases in their life cycle, they share certain elements in common: the disorder flares up during periods of exceptional stress, such as the death of a loved one, illness, loss, or any major change that shakes the foundation of how a woman defines herself. Transitions and ruptures in one's life often set the stage for eating disorders. These are the times to seek support from compassionate friends and family rather than food. Isolation with pastry should be replaced by intimacy with people!

After my father died, I became self-critical about not exercising as regularly as I used to. In my mind, it didn't matter that in addition to my own on-going professional responsibilities, I now had to move my mother to an assisted living facility, clean out the home where I grew up, put the house on the market, and manage my mother's finances, medical appointments, and emotional security. All I could think about is that I wasn't working out and I was going to gain weight. Fortunately, as a psychotherapist, I was able to successfully analyze myself! Faced with the hard and painful truth that my beloved father was never coming back and that my mother was declining as well, I felt powerless, bereft, overwhelmed, and out-of-control. And so I began to fixate on something I could control: my exercise regime. I recruited my body to divert me from the emotional hurt of my heart.

I decided the best way to be "my own best therapist" was to grant myself a grace period to be imperfect. Just because I did not have the time or energy to exercise the way I had, did not mean I couldn't make a partial commitment to exercise. It did not have to be all or nothing. I also sadly recognized that the strain caused by my mother's increased need for my time and care would not last forever. Reminding myself that I wanted to be the best daughter possible to her during this difficult time enabled me to put some of my needs on the back burner, knowing I would return to taking better care of myself when I could.

In Quest of the Fountain of Youth: The Insanity of Vanity

If only we were chimpanzees! A study discovered that male chimpanzees prefer to pair off with an older female rather than find a lady chimp their own age.[54] So strong is the male urge to find an older partner that fights frequently break out over rights of access to the oldest female chimps in the tribe. Although scientists are not sure why this happens, the study suggests that the preference of human men for youthful women may be a recent evolutionary phenomenon. (Who says we are the more evolved species?)

By 2020, more than a third of all Americans will be 50 or older. In this decade, the number of Americans over 65 will surpass the number of Americans under age 20. The quest for the fountain of youth, providing perfect and eternal beauty, has become a national obsession. Cosmetic surgery is now a $15 billion a year industry.

The American Society for Plastic and Reconstructive Surgery

classifies small breasts as a deformity, thus rendering a normal body part as diseased and requiring medical treatment. The normal body changes of aging are now pathologized with labels that sound like illness: our laugh lines are called "nasolabial folds," the fine lines around the lips, "perioral rhytids," and lines between the eyebrows, "glabellar wrinkles."[55]

If you have middle-aged "toe obesity," doctors offer the "foot facelift," which will reduce your toes. You can also have collagen injected into the soles of your feet so your older feet can withstand the daily pounding shock of high heels. (Manolo Blahniks and Jimmy Choo shoes can boast heels of five inches and up).[56]

Hand lifts for older women are now the rage. "The hands are a hot new area," trumpets a New York plastic surgeon who describes the procedure: "Fraxel laser to remove diffuse wrinkling, Thermage for skin tightening, sclerotherapy to treat varicose veins in the hands by injecting a solution into the veins, the Q-switched laser to blast away pigment spots, and injections of fat to plump up the hands."

Not happy with your thinning eyelashes? Try eyelash transplants. Hair follicles are harvested from the back of the scalp and sewn onto the eyelid. The only problem is you now have the extra chore of trimming them, as they will continue to grow.

Plastic surgeons can also enhance your drooping belly button, enlarge your nipples, and even restore your private parts to a tighter, more youthful, rejuvenated appearance. Web sites advertise "designer vaginas." With a tighter vagina, you can now claim to be a "born-again virgin."

Then there's a new procedure to relocate fat from one part of your body to another. (The ultimate in recycling!) New York public relations executive Peggy Siegal explained: "The older you get, the more the fat gravitates to your butt. The doctor takes it out of your bottom and puts it back in your face. So when you are kissing my face, you are actually kissing my [you know what]."[57]

To revitalize your older self, you can also join a surgery safari to Latin America. A friend recently described a vacation to Mexico, where she observed groups of middle-aged American women wandering around town, their faces encased in white turbans, white bandages, and sunglasses. They looked like escapees from a leper colony heading to their Lepers Anonymous group, she laughed.

According to Toni Bentley, a former dancer with the New York City Ballet, "At its most extreme, this craze for plastic surgery is more than a display of culturally conditioned self-hatred. It is, rather, a current manifestation of female masochism—a sister compulsion to anorexia, bulimia, cutting and excessive tattooing and piercing."[58]

And then there is the other extreme school called the "self-inflicted Botox" method to prevent wrinkles. Its mission statement to women is simple: "Reduce all smiling, frowning, or making any facial expression that will promote wrinkles."[59]

There is nothing wrong in trying to look better. Getting rid of a wrinkle here and there may be helpful for self-esteem. Indeed, my friend Renee from high school—now a middle-aged woman—never regretted having her nose job. She claims it improved her appearance and gave her a feeling of self-confidence she did not previously have.

The question becomes: At what point does the desire for plastic surgery turn addictive and become a symptom of body image anxieties? At what point is a woman externalizing her inner unhappiness in hopes that revamping her outside self will remedy her inner dissatisfaction?

Conquering the Inner Terrorist

While we worry about defeating world terrorism, we give little thought to defeating our "inner terrorist" who attacks, condemns, and ridicules our very own body. Many women declare war on their bodies every day. For most women, there is one particular part of the body where their "badness" resides. One self-critical middle-aged woman,

Paula, claimed during an initial therapy consultation that she hated every part of her body. "Every part?" I asked with dismay. "Well, no," Paula conceded, "my wrists are OK." What a small, insignificant part of one's body to like, I thought. How stingy with herself. And how sad.[60]

Paula's approval of only one small part of her body reminds me of Cindy Jackson, who holds the Guinness World Record for cosmetic procedures—52 of them. In Cindy's case, only her dimples remain original.

When a person becomes consumed with self-critical thoughts about her body, it sometimes is a symptom of depression. Unable to find relief from deep internal sadness, she attempts to comfort herself by altering her outer appearance. Women may recruit their bodies to express what they cannot express in words. The body becomes a vehicle to communicate matters of the heart that have no other channel. We crystallize all our emotional pain into one concrete problem: "I hate my aging body. I need to change it, and change it, and change it some more."

In *The Good Body*, Eve Ensler describes her obsession with her "imperfect" stomach. She explains: "I have bought into the idea that if my stomach were flat, then I would be good . . . I would be accepted, admired, important, loved. Maybe because for most of my life I have felt . . . bad, and my stomach is the carrier, the pouch for all that self-hatred. Because my stomach has become the repository for my sorrow, my childhood scars, my unfulfilled ambition, my unexpressed rage. Like a toxic dump . . . My stomach has become my tormentor, my distractor, it's my most serious committed relationship. I've tried to sedate it, educate it, embrace it, and most of all, erase it."[61]

Women tend to be more self-critical of their bodies than men. As Susan Sontag, the critic and feminist, wrote in the essay "The Double Standard of Aging:" "Most men experience getting older with regret, apprehension. But most women experience it even more painfully: with shame."[62]

In her bestselling book, *I Feel Bad About My Neck and Other Thoughts on Being a Woman*, Nora Ephron notes, "Sometimes I think that not having to worry about your hair anymore is the secret upside of death." And, "Anything you think is wrong with your body at the age of 35 you will be nostalgic for at the age of 45."[63]

How Can Older Women Declare Peace with Their Body Image?

So I wonder, as we grow older, is there any hope we may finally declare peace with our bodies? When I read that 90-year-old Helen Gurley Brown, the influential, long-time editor of *Cosmopolitan* magazine, was still doing 200 sit-ups a day until she died, it makes me doubtful. I hope at age 90 I'm not compelled to do 200 sit-ups every day. I'd rather be lying on a tropical beach, reading a mystery novel, drinking a piña colada and feeling totally carefree about the calories!

Jamie Lee Curtis said, "The more I like me, the less I want to pretend to be other people."

Reese Witherspoon said: "Sexuality and femininity is an accumulation of age and wisdom and comfort in your own skin."

Demi Moore, at age 50, admitted, "I have had a love–hate relationship with my body. When I'm at the greatest odds with my body, it's usually because I feel my body's betraying me . . . struggling with my weight and feeling that I couldn't eat what I wanted to eat. . . . I think I sit today in a place of greater acceptance of my body You can't look at yourself in the mirror and tear your body apart. You have to look at it and go, 'Thank you. Thank you for standing by me, for being there for me no matter what I have put you through.'"

In *Sex and the Seasoned Woman: Pursuing the Passionate Life*, Gail Sheehy reflects, "What makes a seasoned woman? Time. A seasoned woman is spicy. She has been marinated in life experience. Like a complex wine, she can be alternately sweet, tart, sparkling, mellow. She is both maternal and playful. Assured, alluring, and resourceful.

The seasoned woman knows who she is. She could be any one of us, as long as she is committed to living fully and passionately in the second half of her life, despite failures and false starts."[64]

While we are continuing to marinate in our life experiences, let's remember there are infinite ways for older women to be beautiful:

- We are more than just our bodies—we have become more knowledgeable, more self-sufficient, wiser, and more empathic to the foibles of the human condition, including our own.
- We can develop our own unique style and flair as older women, independent of what the designers dictate as the latest skinny fashion. The Red Hat Society leads the way, with members dressing in purple dresses and red hats to celebrate middle age with verve, humor, and élan. This is a global society that supports and encourages women in their pursuit of fun, friendship, freedom, fulfillment, and fitness.[65]
- Exercise and keeping fit are key ingredients in helping older women feel at peace with their bodies. Physical activity provides a measure of pride, health, and well-being. We can find new ways of moving—dancing, yoga, stretching, or water aerobics—that enhance our enjoyment of our bodies.
- Be sensuous. Be sexual. It's never too late.
- Discover a new challenge that stimulates you in ways other than fixating on your physical appearance: learn a new language, join a dance class, a book club, a theater group. Middle-aged waists may be expanding, but so can our horizons be expanding![66]

The ultimate truth, of course, is that life is an inside job. How can you commit to living life fully and passionately, despite your weight, your eating, and your sensitivities about aging? Emily Dickinson encouragingly wrote, "We turn not older with years, but newer every day."

"Be bold and love your body. Stop fixing it. It was never broken," declares Eve Ensler.

1 Adapted from Mary Anne Cohen, *French Toast for Breakfast* (Gürze Books, 1995), 17–18.

2 Marlene Boskind-White and William C. White, Jr., *Bulimia/Anorexia: The Binge-Purge Cycle and Self-Starvation* (W. W. Norton, 2001).

3 Because anorexia is the psychiatric disorder with the highest mortality rate, urgent efforts to better understand this illness have resulted in some unusual and odd studies. This research illustrate how much scientists are attempting to leave no stone unturned to get to the bottom of why people want to starve themselves.

The *British Journal of Psychiatry* reports that people born in the spring (from March through June) are more likely to suffer from anorexia. The mother's reduced exposure to sunlight and the subsequent drop in Vitamin D levels during a winter pregnancy appear to contribute to the development of the child's anorexia. G. Disanto, A. E. Handel, A. E. Para, S. V. Ramagopalan, L. Handunnetthi, "Season of Birth and Anorexia Nervosa." *The British Journal of Psychiatry*, May 5, 2011.

"Fingerology"—the study of finger lengths, also known as digit ratio—is being studied by researchers across the globe to predict a variety of addictions and psychiatric disorders. The psychiatry clinic at the University of Erlangen-Nuremberg in Germany has discovered that women whose index finger is shorter than the ring finger are prone to higher levels of anorexia and bulimia. This disparity in finger size is caused by increased amount of testosterone the fetus receives in the womb (*New York Post*, August 28, 2011). Stephanie Jane Quinton, April Rose Smith, Thomas Joiner, "The 2nd to 4th Digit Ratio (2d:4d) and Eating Disorder Diagnosis in Women," *Personality and Individual Differences*, September 2011, vol. 51, 402–405.

The *New York Times* health section reports that "most medical experts agree that a third of people with anorexia will remain chronically ill, a third will die of their disorder, and a third will recover. But there is surprising little agreement as to what 'recovery' means for people with anorexia." Abby Ellin, "In Fighting Anorexia, Recovery Is Elusive" *New York Times*, April 26, 2011.

4 The psychiatric diagnosis of anorexia nervosa (DSM-5) includes a person who: Refuses to maintain normal body weight.

Fears gaining weight or becoming fat, even though he/she is underweight.

Distorts his/her body weight, size, or shape and denies the seriousness of current low body weight.

The change in the diagnosis of anorexia nervosa in the 2013 DSM-5 was to remove the criterion of amenorrhea (loss of menstrual cycle). Removing this criterion means that boys and men with anorexia will be able to receive an appropriate diagnosis. Also, girls and women who continue to have their period, despite other symptoms associated with anorexia, such as weight loss and food restriction, are eligible for a diagnosis of anorexia. In addition, the original criterion for anorexia, that the "patient must be 85% or less than their recommended body weight," is removed. The DSM-5 addresses weight by requiring "restriction of energy intake . . . leading to significantly low body weight."

Between 1 and 5 percent of the population of the United States suffers from anorexia; 90 percent are female and 10 percent male. Statistics show that between 5 and 20 percent of anorexics die because of medical complications due to self-starvation. Starvation can lead to liver, heart, or kidney damage as well as osteoporosis, anemia, depressed immune system, and endocrine abnormalities.

I prefer to use the term "the person with anorexia" to imply that the person is not solely her disease. Anorexia is only one part of her whole self. However, for economy of space, I will use the term anorexic from here on.

Although both males and females may suffer from anorexia, the majority are women, so I have used the feminine pronoun.

A supportive teaching video on anorexia can be viewed online: www.youtube.com/watch?v=ob7puaEM4P8

5   Hilde Bruch, *Eating Disorders: Obesity, Anorexia, and the Person Within* (Basic Books, 1973), 3, 4, 50.

6   In the profession of psychotherapy, increasing value is placed on the therapist's creative use of self—using her own thoughts, feelings, and body sensations to understand the nonverbal world of the patient. Thomas Ogden, *Projective Identification and Psychotherapeutic Technique* (Jason Aronson, 2005), 72.

7   Many doctors believe that anorexics can have physical recovery but often remain chronically preoccupied with food and weight and vulnerable to relapse under stress. Others believe a full restoration of nutritional, physical, emotional, and psychological health is possible. Abby Ellin, "In Fighting Anorexia, Recovery Is Elusive" *New York Times*, April 26, 2011.

Girls with anorexia seek each other out on the Internet looking for support for their self- starvation. This community encourages their drive to starve themselves. A selection of user names on "The Hunger Blogs" paints a vivid picture of the inner preoccupation of the anorexic: Cursesatmirrors, coffeeandhipbones, featherweightgirl, carvingoutcollarbones, thewinneristhethinner, iwillbethinandperfect. Although Internet service providers commit to shutting down these sites, they continue to mushroom.

8   D.M. Garner and P.E. Garfinkel, eds., *Handbook of Psychotherapy for Anorexia Nervosa and Bulimia* (Guilford Press, 1985) 75.

9   Hilde Bruch, *Eating Disorders: Obesity, Anorexia, and the Person Within.*

10   In 1944, the Swiss psychiatrist Ludwig Binswanger chronicled his treatment of Ellen West. Ludwig Binswanger, "The Case of Ellen West: An Anthropological-Clinical Study," in Rollo May, Ernest Angel, and Henri F. Ellenberger, eds., *Existence: A New Dimension in Psychiatry and Psychology* (Basic Books, 1958), 237–364.

11   Bulimia nervosa as defined in the DSM-5:
Recurrent episodes of binge eating, followed by an attempt to rid oneself of the food. A feeling of lack of control over eating behavior during the eating binges.
Binges are usually followed by purging.
    A minimum average of at least one binge/purge episode a week for three months.
    Self-worth for the bulimic is strongly influenced by body shape and weight.
    Bulimia is divided into the purging or non-purging type. Purging methods include self-induced vomiting and overuse of laxatives, diuretics, or enemas. The nonpurging bulimic goes on fasts or strict diets or engages in excessive exercise to prevent weight gain.
    Prior to 2013, the diagnosis for bulimia nervosa included "at least two binge/purge episodes a week for three months."
    Like the other eating disorders anorexia and compulsive overeating, bulimia is more frequent in females than males. However, there are many more male bulimics than male anorexics.

12   Sharon Farber, Ph.D., *When the Body Is the Target* (Rowman & Littlefield, 2000). A rich resource on self-harm and eating disorders that explores the connection with early family attachment problems.

13   Sharon Farber, *When the Body Is the Target,* 231.

14   Joyce McDougall, *Theaters of the Body: A Psychoanalytic Approach to Psychosomatic Illness* (W.W. Norton, 1989).

15   Jane Brody, "The Growing Wave of Teenage Self-Injury," *New York Times,* May 6, 2008; http://www.nytimes.com/learning/teachers/featured_articles/20080506tuesday.html
    The singer Demi Lovato, age 19, vividly describes the connection between her depression, anxiety, and self-cutting in *Self* magazine (August 2012): "There were times I felt so anxious, almost like I was crawling out of my skin—that if I didn't do something physical to match the way I felt inside, I would explode. I cut myself to take my mind off that."

16   Mary Anne Cohen, *French Toast for Breakfast: Declaring Peace with Emotional Eating*. (Gürze Books, 1995), chapter 10, "Medication, Mood, and Mallomars."

17   "Addicted to Sweat" is the name of Madonna's 2013 DVD. Madonna begins her punishing daily routine with a three-hour session of Ashtanga yoga, followed by a Pilates session before lunch. She then alternates her third daily session between karate, pumping iron, running, swimming, cycling, and occasionally horseback riding.
     The physical effects of intense workouts and exercise addiction can clearly be seen in celebrities who seem to be all skin and veins: Donna McConnell, "Skin and veins: Celebrity gym-addicts whose love of exercise is spoiling their looks," March 5, 2008, *Daily Mail;* http://www.dailymail.co.uk/tvshowbiz/article-525768/Skin-veins-Celebrity-gym-addicts-love-exercise-spoiling-looks.html#ixzz2OTKaw1UX.

18   The DSM-5 adds Binge Eating Disorder (BED) as a separate diagnosis; it had previously been classified under the more general diagnosis of Eating Disorder Not Otherwise Specified (EDNOS). BED is defined as having "a sense of lack of control over eating," with the person suffering also exhibiting three or more of the following:

> Frequent episodes of eating large amounts of food more rapidly than normal.
> Eating large amounts of food when not feeling physically hungry.
> Feeling out of control with the quantity of food eaten.
> Bingeing, often followed by stomach pain, sleepiness, or uncomfortable fullness.
> Shame or guilt over eating/weight.
> Depression, isolation, anxiety disorders, or low self-esteem.
> Eating alone because of shame about how much one is eating.
> Episodic dieting; dieting believed to be a solution to problems.

     BED may be the most common eating disorder affecting, as much as 3 percent of the U.S. population, or roughly 10 million Americans, three times more than those diagnosed with anorexia and bulimia combined. BED also has significant medical complications. Those suffering with BED will benefit by having a separate diagnostic category, because they will now receive the proper diagnosis and treatment.

19   A Swiss woman starved to death. A follower of Breatharianism, she believed she could survive on light alone. *New York Post*, April 26, 2012, 9.

20   Debra Waterhouse, *Why Women Need Chocolate: Eat What You Crave to Look Good and Feel Great* (Diane Publishing Company, 1995), 42. Emphasis added.

21   Jan Chozen Bays, M.D., *Mindful Eating: A Guide to Rediscovering a Healthy and Joyful Relationship with Food* (Shambala, 2009).

22   According to the National Association to Advance Fat Acceptance (NAAFA), 65 million Americans are labeled obese. The United States Centers for Disease

Control estimates that in 2009–2010, 35.7 percent of all Americans are obese: http://www.cdc.gov/obesity/data/adult.html. In 2009–2010, the prevalence of obesity was 35.5% among adult men and 35.8% among adult women. K.M. Flegal et al., "Prevalence of Obesity and Trends in the Distribution of Body Mass Index Among Us Adults, 1999–2010," *Journal of the American Medical Association*, February 2012, vol. 307, 491–497; http://jama.ama assn.org/content/early/2012/01/20/jama.2012.39.abstract.

23   Glen Gaesser, *Big Fat Lies: The Truth About Your Weight and Your Health* (Gürze Books, 2002), 59.

24   J.L. Kuk et al., "Edmonton Obesity Staging System: Association with Weight History and Mortality Risk," *Applied Physiology, Nutrition, and Metabolism*, volume 36, August 2011, 570–576.

25   Gina Kolata, "Brown Fat, Triggered by Cold or Exercise, May Yield a Key to Weight Control," *New York Times*, January 24, 2012; http://www.nytimes.com/2012/01/25/health/brown-fat-burns-ordinary-fat-study-finds.html?_r=0.

26   A. Andersen, L. Cohn, and T. Holbrook, *Making Weight: Healing Men's Conflicts with Food, Weight, Shape and Appearance* (Gürze Books, 2000), 140.
A person's size is 70 percent determined by genes. Two overweight parents = 90 percent chance of becoming obese; one obese birth parent = 40 percent chance of obesity.
Tara Pope-Parker, "When Fatty Feasts Are Driven by Automatic Pilot," *New York Times*, July 11, 2011; http://well.blogs.nytimes.com/2011/07/11/when-fatty-feasts-are-driven-by-automatic-pilot/?scp=1&sq=When%20Fatty%20Feasts%20are%20driven%20by%20automatic%20pilot&st=cse.

27   A. Andersen, *Making Weight*, 136.

28   The Web site www.naafa.org is a rich resource of self-help and advocacy.

29   For more information: www.Overeatersanonymous.org.

30   The American Society for Metabolic and Bariatric Surgery has helpful information on its web site: www.asmbs.org.

31   For more on the risks and benefits of weight-loss surgery, see http://www.mayoclinic.com/health/gastric-bypass/MY00825.

32   More on the risks of weight-loss surgery: http://www.thinnertimes.com/weight-loss-surgery/gastric-bypass/gastric-bypass-complications.html.

33   Linda Bacon, Ph.D., *Health at Every Size: The Surprising Truth About Your Weight* (BenBella Books, 2010). See also the Health at Every Size Web site: www. haescommunity.org.

34   *Men's Health*, November 2011. Teenage boys are suffering increased anxiety about body image and are more willing to engage in risky behaviors: Douglas Quenqua, "Muscular Body Image Lures Boys Into Gym, and Obsession," *New York Times*, November 19, 2012; http://www.nytimes.com/2012/11/19/health/teenage-boys-worried-about-body-image-take-risks.html?nl=todaysheadlines&emc=edit_th_20121119. Marla E. Eisenberg, et al., "Muscle-enhancing Behaviors Among Adolescent Girls and Boys," *Pediatrics*, December 2012, vol. 130, no. 6; http://pediatrics.aappublications.org/content/early/2012/11/14/peds.2012-0095.abstract.

35   Rising machismo is not limited to America and western Europe. "Scholars note that the body images of some Hindu deities, especially the god of Ram, have undergone a re-imagining during the past two decades. Before, Ram was often depicted as lithe and slender, but by the 1990s artists were usually depicting him as a muscular deity. Many calendar artists told scholars that they altered the image to succeed in a changed marketplace." Jim Yardley, "A Quest for Six-Packs, Inspired by Bollywood," *New York Times*, July 18, 2012; http://www.nytimes.com/2012/07/19/world/asia/on-screen-abdominals-send-indias-men-to-gym.html?ref=world.

36   Susan Albers, Psy.D., "Manorexia," *Psychology Today*, May 10, 2010; http://www.psychologytoday.com/blog/comfort-cravings/201005/manorexia.
    The director of a J. Crew clothing shop in Manhattan has observed the intense interest the "manorexic" guy has in fashion. He declares, "Men are the new women." (I shudder and hope he's wrong!) James B. Stewart, "The Rise of Men in Suits. Slim Ones," *New York Times*, November 23, 2012; http://www.nytimes.com/2012/11/24/business/slim-suits-help-lead-gains-in-mens-wear.html?pagewanted=all.

37   David Colman, "Manorexic Models," *New York Magazine*, May 2, 2010; http://nymag.com/news/intelligencer/topic/65753/.

38   The United States Army is investigating whether certain dietary supplements for athletes, available until recently on military bases in the U.S., may have played a role in the deaths of two soldiers. The article quotes the product description of one of the supplements, "gives you the mad aggressive desire and ability to lift more weight, pump out more reps and have crazy lasting energy." Peter Lattman and Natasha Singer, "Army Studies Workout Supplements After Deaths," *New York Times*, February 2, 2012; http://www.nytimes.com/2012/02/03/business/army-studies-workout-supplements-after-2-deaths.html.

39   Ron Saxen, *Good Eater: The True Story of One Man's Struggle with Binge Eating Disorder* (New Harbinger Publications, 2007).

40   Roni Caryn Rabin, "Men Struggle for Rape Awareness," *New York Times*, January 23, 2012; http://www.nytimes.com/2012/01/24/health/as-victims-men-struggle-for-rape-awareness.html?pagewanted=all.

41   MaleSurvivor.Org is a national group committed to healing and preventing the sexual victimization of men and boys. The organization offers online and in-person discussion forums and conferences. The organization serves the community of men who have been victimized, their significant others, and mental health professionals.

42   *Do I Look Fat*, a 2005 film by Travis Mathews; www.doilookfatthemovie.com.

43   National Eating Disorders.Org: http://www.nationaleatingdisorders.org/neda-Dir/files/documents/handouts/MalesRes.pdf. The National Association for Males with Eating Disorders offers a comprehensive web site regarding causes, treatment, and personal stories of men in recovery from eating disorders: www.namedinc.org.

44   Adriana Lima, the Victoria's Secret supermodel, quickly got into shape after the birth of her second child. The *New York Times* reported the herculean efforts she exerted to accomplish this: Adriana worked out with her coach "six hours a day, seven days a week for five weeks." Courtney Rubin, "Getting Models Into Fighting Shape," *New York Times*, February 7, 2012; http://www.nytimes.com/2013/02/07/fashion/getting-models-into-fighting-shape.html?_r=0.

45   Tara Parker-Pope, "During Pregnancy, Starving for Two," *New York Times*, June 2, 2009; http://well.blogs.nytimes.com/2009/06/02/starving-for-twoa/.

46   S.J. Crow et al., "Eating Disorder Symptoms in Pregnancy: A Prospective Study," *International Journal of Eating Disorders*, 2008, vol. 41, 277–279.

47   Jane Brody, "Life in Womb May Affect Adult Heart Disease Risk," *New York Times*, October 1, 1996.

48   Judith Viorst, *How Did I Get to Be 40* (Simon & Schuster, 1976).

49   *New Beauty Magazine*, Spring-Summer 2011, volume 7, issue 2.

50   Maria Russo, "Farewell to Youth, but Not Beauty," *New York Times*, March 1, 2012; http://www.nytimes.com/2012/03/04/fashion/older-women-are-the-new-faces-of-beauty.html?pagewanted=all.

51   Marianne Schnall, "Jane Fonda on Men, Power and Plastic Surgery," *Glamour,* February 1, 2007; http://www.glamour.com/magazine/2007/02/jane-fonda.

52   Quentin Letts, "Camilla," *Wall Street Journal,* November 5, 2005; http://online.wsj.com/article/SB113115020324588993.html.

53   Maureen Dowd, *Are Men Necessary: When Sexes Collide* (Berkley Books, 2006).

54   Martin N. Muller, Melissa Emery Thompson, Richard W. Wrangham, "Male Chimpanzees Prefer Mating with Old Females," *Current Biology,* November 21, 2006, 2234–2238.

55   Sander Gilman, *Making the Body Beautiful: A Cultural History of Aesthetic Surgery* (Princeton University Press, 2001).

56   "Dangerous Elegance: A History of High-Heeled Shoes," http://www.randomhistory.com/1-50/036heels.html.

57   Alex Kuszynski, *Beauty Junkies: Inside Our $15 Billion Obsession With Cosmetic Surgery* (Broadway Books, 2008).

58   Toni Bentley, "Nip and Tuck," *New York Times* Sunday Book Review, October 22, 2006.

59   Stylelist.com, November 12, 2011.

60   In an article in the *Daily News* on April 21, 2013, entitled, "How Terrorists Are Born," Mitchell Silber, executive manager director of K2 intelligence and former director of intelligence analysis for the New York Police Department, asks, "What motivates young men to fall down the rabbit hole of radicalism and become terrorists? In most cases, they started out as relatively secular individuals. However, as a result of a lack of strong identity, personal crisis or feelings of alienation, homegrown terrorists develop."
      I believe the dynamics between the "inner terrorist" of the eating disorder person and those who become violent terrorists have striking parallels. Eating disorder people become "radicalized" as they can grow increasingly fanatical about the "Religion of Thinness" and are triggered by similar reasons: "a lack of strong identity, personal crisis or feelings of alienation." The inner terrorist wants to subdue, conquer, and take his/her body hostage in the name of the God of Thinness.

61   Eve Ensler, *The Good Body* (Villard, 2005).

62   Susan Sontag, "The Double Standard of Aging," *The Saturday Review*, September 23, 1972, 29–38.

63   Nora Ephron, *I Feel Bad About My Neck and Other Thoughts on Being a Woman* (Vintage, 2008).

64   Gail Sheehy, *Sex and the Seasoned Woman: Pursuing the Passionate Life.* (Ballantine, 2007).

65   The Red Hat Society (redhatsociety.com) believes "Silliness is the comedy relief of life, and since we are all in it together, we might as well join red-gloved hands and go for the gusto together. Underneath the frivolity, we share a bond of affection, forged by common life experiences and a genuine enthusiasm for wherever life takes us next."

66   A web site from the National Institute on Aging, part of the National Institutes of Health, is devoted to resources for sustaining vibrant health and exercise as an older person: http://go4life.nia.nih.gov//birthday.

4. Bodies and Culture: From Combat to Compassion

Culture, Corsets, and Consciousness

My grandmother's corset, known as "The Contraption," had hooks and eyes, crisscross laces, wire bones with a zipper, and hanging garters. It was made of flesh-colored rubber and encased her from her bosom down to her mid-thighs. As a nine-year-old child I remember watching with fascination and concern as Grandma enclosed herself into "The Contraption" by inhaling, yanking, pulling, tugging, grunting, and sweating. The message I got was that her rounded, full curves were something that needed controlling and taming. At all costs.

Decades later, I am in Louisiana visiting Southern plantations from the 1850s. The plush drawing rooms are furnished with "fainting couches." These couches were designed for the heavily corseted, fashionable women of that era who needed a place to delicately swoon when they lost their breath because their corsets were laced up so tightly.

Who knew that 100 years later, my Eastern European grandmother and the Southern belles like Scarlett O'Hara—with her 17-inch tightly corseted waist—had something in common!

And now, over 50 years since Grandma's "Contraption," I browse a lingerie catalogue offering an "open-bust mid-thigh bodysuit" and panties with "powerful tummy taming panels and mega compression zones" and a "powershape firm control high-waisted thigh smoother."[1]

This tyranny of suffocating one's body spans the generations and stimulates in me a poem:

Ode to Curtailing a Curve

Constrain. Compress. Constrict.
Contract. Control. Contain.
Confine. Conform. Contort.
Contrite.

The media and fashion industries promote perpetual body dissatisfaction so we will buy their self-improvement products. From head to toe, women and men do battle with their bodies.

These messages can set the stage for body discontentment which can contribute to the development of eating disorders:

- A young male patient of mine announces, "I only want a girlfriend who is 'model material.'"
- A girl speaks enviously of her sister, "She's so thin, she's just a dot. If only I could be a size 0 like her, my life would really be great."
- A husband jokes about his wife, who is 15 pounds overweight, "She is pretty from afar, but far from pretty."
- A car bumper sticker jeers, "You're fat and your mother dresses you funny."
- The logo for a gym reads Hard Bodies = Eye Candy.
- An advertisement advises, "The most important decision I ever made was choosing my spouse. The second, my plastic surgeon."
- Actress Cindy Crawford views her digitally altered, airbrushed image and ruefully states, "Even *I* wish I looked like Cindy Crawford."

- An ad for plastic surgery shows a woman with a nose job, promising this procedure helped her live "Happily Ever After."
- The girdle ad suggests, "Think of it [our girdle] as a beautiful alternative to holding your breath." (As if holding your breath is an alternative we should all consider).
- The photo from a Miami magazine shows a very buxom Asian woman. The doctor's ad asks, "Why envy?" indicating that if you too had this woman's breast implants, you would have nothing to ever envy. On the model's hip is a tattoo branded with the doctor's name, "Made by Dr. F.P."
- The *New York Times* describes "Bridal Hunger Games" where brides-to-be, anxious to lose weight before their wedding, have a nasogastric tube inserted from their nose, down the esophagus, to their stomach. This leads to rapid weight loss due to the minimum calories they absorb.[2]
- Oscar Wilde described the capriciousness of style, "Fashion is merely a form of ugliness so unbearable that we are compelled to alter it every six months."

Body preoccupation and apprehensions have become universal. I have treated native-born women and girls from Russia, Argentina, England, Costa Rica, Poland, Peru, Israel, Saint Lucia, Canada, Mexico, France, Puerto Rico, Haiti, Germany, Venezuela, Colombia, England, Cuba, and several Middle Eastern countries. I have spoken with eating disorder therapists from Canada, Mexico, Brazil, and Spain. *The International Journal of Eating Disorders* explores the rise of eating disorders in such far-flung places as Bulgaria, Greece, Iran, Switzerland, Ireland, Mexico, Viet Nam, Australia, and Japan. In 2012 the Iceland Association for Body Acceptance was founded in Reykjavik. All nations and cultures, it seems, are susceptible to eating disorders and body hatred.[3]

The stereotype of a person with an eating disorder is a white, middle- or upper-class girl. Although curvy black women and Latinas traditionally were celebrated and did not experience as much anxiety or shame about their bodies, this has changed significantly.[4] African American, Hispanic, and Asian Americans are now joining the eating disorder population. In some cases, minority men and women believe that being thin will help them assimilate and fit into mainstream white culture.[5]

Racism and discrimination contribute to body distress in sometimes subtle ways. When I was a teenager in the 1960s, certain girls wanted to look less Jewish and had surgery to alter their "Jewish nose." This surgery became all the rage. Renee came to school one Monday morning with a new nose. The following week, Sari appeared with her new nose. Then several months later, in walked Judy with a ski-slope nose almost identical to Renee's and Sari's. New noses were the Sweet 16 presents from their families.

Nose jobs became so popular that it led one rabbi to quip, "You can change your noses, but you can't change your Moses!" In 1923, the Jewish actress, Fanny Brice, had a nose job to avoid being typecast in ethnic roles. The writer Dorothy Parker retorted that Brice "had cut off her nose to spite her *race*."[6]

Elena, a Mexican American young woman, spoke of the pain she felt on receiving her high school graduation photos. "The photographer had airbrushed my nose to look less Mexican and more Anglo. He made my nose thinner and longer, so the picture didn't even look like me. I had never felt there was anything wrong with my nose before. The fact that he just assumed I would like myself better with a white person's nose left me feeling betrayed. I have been bulimic for many years and am now in recovery. I know the experience with the photograph didn't make me bulimic, but it was part of an ongoing message I got as a Latina about not being good enough or pretty enough."[7]

Lorraine, an African American woman, described her struggles with her black skin and nappy hair, "My first experience with racism came from my very own family. My mother, father, and sister have lighter skin than me. My mother never seemed to forgive me for being born with dark skin and kinky hair. She took offense as if I did this to her on purpose, and she tortured me with hair-straightening treatments from a very young age. She also told me to pinch my nose and press my lips together to make them smaller and less black-looking. I determined to marry a black man darker than me so he could never hold my color against me like my mother did. I know there are many reasons for my life-long bingeing disorder and body issues, but these early experiences led me to feel ugly and inadequate."[8]

Once upon a time in the South Pacific Fiji islands, it was a traditional compliment to say, "How beautiful you look. You've gained weight!" But just a few years after the introduction of television in the early 1990s to a province of Fiji's main island, eating disorders—once virtually unheard of there—are on the rise among girls, according to a study presented at the American Psychiatric Association. Three years after Western television came to the region, there was an increase in body dissatisfaction and eating disorders, as young girls began to anxiously obsess about trying to look like the slender, white movie stars of western television.[9]

China has also become a society obsessed with bodies and stature, and remedies to make women taller are big business in that country. Hundreds of young Chinese women are submitting to surgery promising to make them taller. The procedure severs the thighbone. The girl is fitted with metal leg-stretching frames, with pins that pierce the skin and are screwed into the bone. Unfortunately, many of them have experienced a "slight" drawback to this procedure—they can never walk again. So many people were crippled by this surgery that it was finally banned.[10]

In Nairobi, Kenyan women are doing battle with their black skins. Lightening skin creams promote, "the lighter you look, the lovelier you look." However, extended use of these creams can cause a backlash of the skin darkening unevenly, mercury poisoning, or skin cancer.[11]

The Wall Street Journal reported a horrifying practice inflicted on young women in the Arab world called "gavage." Gavage refers to the intentional fattening of teenage girls by force-feeding them in order to heighten their appeal as prospective brides. "In a land such as Mauritania in Africa that suffers from a constant shortage of food, plump women are assumed to be wealthy and more likely to bear children," the article states. Sometimes girls are force-fed to such a degree that their skin tears under the pressure. If they protest this treatment, their toes or fingers are broken by their family to make them eat. This is uncomfortably reminiscent of the technique used by the French to force-feed geese in order to fatten up the goose livers—otherwise known as the delicacy foie gras.[12]

Makeover television shows are blossoming more than ever because they feed into—and add to—the chronic body dissatisfaction of our culture: "Extreme Makeover," "The Swan," "A Makeover Story," "Cosmetic Surgery Before and After," "Queer Eye for the Straight Guy," "The Biggest Loser."

Fortunately, there is some growing awareness of the destructiveness of fashion and body images. *The International Herald Tribune* reports the international fashion industry has been under scrutiny for exalting ultra-thin models on the runways. Criticism became heightened following the deaths of several runway models from self-starvation. The head of the Center on Media and Child Health at Children's Hospital Boston, Dr. Michael Rich, coined the term "eating disorder porn" to describe the emaciated and sexualized models of the Victoria's Secret Fashion Show.

In response, Giorgio Armani urged designers to stop using underweight models, whom he dubbed "human hangers." The owner of an Israeli modeling agency, Adi Barkan, is quoted, "The modeling agencies say, 'Go lose 10 pounds.' But they don't care how the girls do it.

We package malnutrition in such an attractive way that young women everywhere aspire to have 'the look.' It is time this industry shows the world that beauty and high fashion do not equal starvation."[13]

Culture and Body Image Problems

Does the relentless pursuit of thinness portrayed in the fashion world, Hollywood, and advertising *cause* eating disorders? Is our culture responsible for the millions of people who suffer from body image dissatisfaction?

The answer is yes and no. It is true that fashion trends and movie star images create dissatisfaction in the men and women who unfavorably compare themselves. It is true we are bombarded by weight-loss and dieting ads that can make us feel inadequate. It is true anorexia is glamorized and thinness is equated with success. And it is true that looking "hot and sexy" is touted as the key to feeling good about yourself. The obsession to be beautiful and thin provides women with a ready-made identity in an attempt to shore up shaky self-confidence.[14]

However, in spite of the above, culture does not *cause* body hatred. It is only one contributing factor. All of us are exposed to the incessant messages about looking perfect, but not all of us develop body image struggles or eating disorders. Only those with a pre-existing vulnerability tend to internalize these messages in a psychologically self-destructive way. The psychological and biological seeds for an eating disorder and body image disturbance get planted early in a person's life. Pointing to culture as the cause of eating disorders oversimplifies and downplays the emotional complexity and genetic underpinnings of the disorder.

Therapists in the addiction field use the metaphor of a gun to illustrate the origin of an eating disorder. A person's genes, metabolism, and heredity *create* the gun. A troubled or unempathic relationship with one's parents, problems of loss, grief, or abuse, compounded by our culture's relentless pursuit of thinness, *loads* the gun. A specific, emotionally distressful occurrence *pulls* the gun's trigger. An eating disorder then gets activated.

A complicated interaction of factors, such as family stress and heredity, *predisposes* someone to an eating struggle. Then, trauma or loss *precipitates* an eating disorder, while unresolved grief or addiction *perpetuates* the eating behavior.[15]

The emotionally distressful occurrence that pulls the gun's trigger varies, of course, from person to person. The trigger, however, is usually a disruption, transition, or loss that feels unsettling or dangerous to the person's emotional equilibrium: puberty, a death, divorce, sexual or physical abuse, going away to college, moving, an illness, retirement. These events threaten one's self esteem, create anxiety, and leave a person feeling uprooted. In attempting to regain control of what feels like an out-of-control situation, the person displaces her fears by going on a diet to lose weight, which she believes will somehow "solve" the upset. Dieting is about controlling and regulating. It is often the first step that sets in motion the vicious cycle of food restriction, leading to bingeing, and then purging. As we try harder and harder to take charge of our life, the eating disorder moves in. Our focus diverts from the emotional threat we are suffering and shifts onto trying to lose weight and make our bodies perfect.

Food for Thought: Confronting Cultural Messages

To heal our internal struggles, we need to study the personal, psychological dynamics that create our body dissatisfaction. All true healing begins with the human heart. But we also need to confront the cultural messages infiltrating our psyches that contribute to making us feel bad about ourselves. The goal of advertising is to promote our dissatisfaction about how we look so we will buy more products to allegedly improve our appearance.

Observe

Observe how many advertisements for cars, credit cards, cigarettes, liquors, and power tools utilize a sexy, young female body to sell their product. Observe how many ads prey upon women's and men's insecurity around sexual appeal, weight, hair, odor, and fashion to sell their products. Observe how many actresses and models have impossibly flawless skin, hair, figures. There is never any cellulite nor blemish nor stray hair, because these images have been photoshopped. It has been said that striving for perfection turns you into a failure even before you begin!

A patient of mine, struggling to resolve a binge eating disorder and make peace with her larger body, worked in the industry that digitally alters photographs of female models for magazine displays. She, more than anyone, was aware of the falsity and fantasy that goes into constructing this ideal perfect female. And yet she too fought against the impulse to buy into the message that achieving perfection through weight loss is simply a matter of willpower and, if you just try harder, you will finally be happy and self-accepting.

Critique and Question

Share your observations with your friends and family. Today I saw a newspaper advertisement for bathroom tiles showing the backsides of two females in bikinis. Female buttocks selling marble tiles? The connection eludes me. I think they have their ad campaign ass backward!

The sexualization of young girls is also frightening and lamentable and deserves critiquing. Thong underwear for young girls, padded bikini tops (starting at age seven), high heels on two-year-olds, Halloween costumes looking suspiciously like stripper outfits, are all an "approved" version of child pornography. Child beauty contests showcase girls with makeup, wigs, false eyelashes, and sexy outfits way beyond their years. The program "Toddlers and Tiaras" recently presented a four-year-old girl all decked out with fake breasts and fake padding on her backside.[16]

Accept

Genetics are responsible for a large percentage of your body shape. Small breasts, balding heads, ample backsides, even metabolism all have a genetic component. You cannot change your genes, no matter how much you starve, diet, or exercise. Everybody has a "set point," the weight range that your body always seeks to return to, no matter how much you diet or exercise. This genetic pull is hard to evade.

Appreciate

You may not love everything about your body—maybe far from it. Yet this is the body that takes you places, makes love, makes babies, dances, goes on vacation, and cooperates with you in so many ways so you can partake in the satisfactions of life. Recognize that the people you love most in the world all have imperfections. And you don't love them any less!

My grandmother, with those soft round curves, was delicious for hugging and cuddling when she took off "The Contraption" at the end of the day.

From Combat to Compassion

Though we travel the world over to find the beautiful, we must carry it with us or we find it not.

—Ralph Waldo Emerson

"Mirror, mirror on the wall, who's the fairest of them all?" asks Snow White's stepmother and countless women as they gaze anxiously at their faces and their bodies. Rare is the woman who responds, "Me!

I'm the fairest in the land (or at least one of the contenders)!"

Too often, the feedback we perceive from the mirror is warped, critical, fragmented, and negative.

The first "mirror" in our lives is our mother's gaze when we were a baby. Her gaze reflects back to us if she finds us lovable and is happy about our birth. A mother who is self-preoccupied, chronically depressed, anxious, critical, or ambivalent about having a child will present a warped mirror to her child. Her eyes and face will not shine lovingly as she looks upon her child. The baby perceives this as she gazes at her mother's face and does not feel reassured that she is special. Thus begin issues of self-esteem and body image disturbance.[17]

What Is Body Image?

Body image refers to the inner thoughts, feelings, attitudes, and judgments we have about our appearance, as well as what we imagine other people think about our looks. Body image is not necessarily a realistic, objective perception but rather the *mental* image we carry inside ourselves—distortions and all. Because our body image is colored by our emotions and moods, it is psychological in nature. It can fluctuate from moment to moment. We may wake up one morning feeling positive, only to be immediately deflated once we step on the scale and see weight gain. Or we may like an outfit we are wearing, only to be deflated as our mother looks us over and rolls her eyes in disapproval.

Most of us have some measure of body image distortion. We may overestimate how fat we are, how big our nose is, how puny our muscles are. Anorexics are most known for suffering from severe body image distortion. The anorexic clamors about how unbearably fat she is as her family looks on with disbelief and horror at her increasing emaciation.

Early in my career, I asked Zoe, a 15-year-old anorexic girl, to draw what she thought were the contours of her body on a blank six-foot-square paper I had taped on my office wall. The silhouette she outlined was almost three times her real size.

In the hope of injecting a note of reality, I asked Zoe if she would allow me to trace her outline as she stood against the paper. The divergence between my realistic drawing and Zoe's imagined shape caused her tremendous agitation. She could not believe nor accept the discrepancy. I quickly realized that Zoe *emotionally* needed to see herself as a very large girl. My demonstrating the truth to her only made her feel more disturbed. Not my intention! I never used that exercise again. Instead, I now empathically seek to understand the *psychological* meaning of feeling fat for each person I work with.

Concerns about body image effect different people in different ways. One woman goes on vacation and may regret she didn't exercise more during the year, but still puts on a bathing suit, hops into the ocean and enjoys herself anyway. Her body image concerns have not gotten in the way of her pleasure. Another woman, with a similar body and less self-confidence, may sit on the beach all covered up, too embarrassed, miserable, and self-conscious to disrobe and go swimming.[18]

Because a person is attractive does not guarantee she or he will have a good body image. As a beginning therapist 40 years ago at a mental health clinic, I treated an extraordinarily beautiful patient who was also schizophrenic. She heard inner destructive voices that impaired her ability to function in her everyday life. And yet, I must confess, a part of me could not understand why her beauty did not conquer her mental illness. I naively believed at that time, like so many women, "How could anyone so gorgeous have any problems at all?" Experience has indeed taught me otherwise.

Models and actors—no matter how attractive they may realistically be—are often notorious for their self-hatred and suffer from rampant eating disorders. Two exceedingly attractive patients of mine—one a professional fashion model and the other a 20-year-old Sophia Loren lookalike—were beset by body hatred and out-of-control eating disorders. Their outward beauty could not triumph over their *inner* distorted sense of ugliness. We discovered that their inability to feel good about their appearance was based on the emotional residue of childhood traumatic abuse experiences. Both women had been physically and sexually abused as children. To move forward in their lives, they needed to confront their trauma, grieve the betrayal, and reclaim ownership over their own bodies.

What Is a Healthy Body Image?

A person with a healthy body image maintains a flexible attitude and a realistic perspective about the normal variations of his or her body. In other words, if you gained a couple of pounds over the weekend, it doesn't mean you are now fat and ugly for the rest of your life. Or, if you neglected to work out last week, it doesn't mean your muscles have atrophied and you look like the skinny kid from when you were ten years old.

A healthy body image does not mean you have to love every part of your body without reservation. It means that, for the most part, you can live peacefully in your own skin. A flexible body image takes into account that women often get bloated when premenstrual. It also means they gain weight when pregnant and need to tolerate living in a larger body for a while. It means accepting that as people age they do have more wrinkles, less muscle tone, and often gain weight. These are normal stages of body development.

A healthy body image means you are more than the sum of your physical parts—that you have an *integrated* sense of your body, mind, and spirit, rather than feeling persecuted by a particular body part. It also means your physical appearance is *not* the only measure of your happiness and worth. Your sense of self is influenced not just by your looks but by the loving relationships in your life, your productive work, the ability to be playful, and your spiritual sense of nature and the universe.

Body Dissatisfaction

Despite the movie *Real Women Have Curves* and a recent book, *Men Prefer Curves*, and a woman's health club named Curves, many women are in constant battle with their curves, their appetites, and their bodies.

Beset by chronic worry and dissatisfaction with their bodies, women and men engage in a multitude of ways to modify their offending body part(s). The range of body manipulation methods extends along a continuum from benign to highly dangerous. Noninvasive methods include exercising, diet, makeup, or dying one's hair. Invasive methods include body piercing, tattoos, laxatives and diet pills, liposuction, and plastic surgery.

The media is replete with articles on how often women and girls alter their bodies in the hopes of finally feeling good about themselves. Girls are having breast implants at increasingly younger ages, while women are subjecting themselves to Botox injections, liposuction, breast implants, tummy tucks, hymen "reconstruction" (to become a "born-again" virgin) and the "Barbie" surgery to surgically cut out the inner labia to make the vagina look "nice and tidy" and "prettier."[19]

Each year a new and different body part is targeted for improvement. You can now permanently tattoo eye makeup and lipstick. Or you can focus just on your eyebrows and visit one of the many eyebrow shaping and threading salons that have recently sprouted across the country. Or, if that is not pleasing enough, eyebrow transplants requiring implanting 400 hair follicles from the scalp have seen a rise in demand. Or you can turn your brown eyes permanently blue through laser treatment that removes the patches of brown pigment from the eyes. Or you can surgically slim down your "cankles" (fat calves and ankles). Or you can have an operation that sculpts your foot so you can show "toe cleavage" in your sexy high heels. Even your navel is not exempt. A recent newspaper story reads, "This year's chic belly button accessory is a scalpel." Since only nonprotruding belly buttons are currently stylish, plastic surgeons will surgically alter your offending belly button for thousands of dollars.

Cosmetic surgery can often be a person's attempt to find an external solution to *internal* anxiety and unhappiness. Some serial cosmetic surgery seekers never alleviate, in a lasting way, their inner cravings to feel good about themselves, no matter how many changes they make to their bodies. Resolving chronic body discomfort is an *inside* job about disentangling emotions, not banishing wrinkles.

Pro-anorexia and pro-bulimia web sites have proliferated on the Internet. They promote self-destructive eating behavior and negative body image by teaching girls that "food is evil," "being thin is more important than being healthy," and "thou shalt not eat without feeling guilty."

As we saw in chapter 3, "Men and Eating Disorders," men are not spared from body dissatisfaction either. Many men experience great dismay and even shame at their loss of hair and increasing baldness. They fear that baldness reveals to the world a loss of physical strength and a waning of sexual prowess. After all, in the Bible, Samson was tremendously virile and, as the song goes, "All his strength was on the top of his head." Men with body image issues often pin various anxieties on losing their hair rather than directly facing worries about competition with other men, sexual adequacy, and concerns about ageing.

In addition, a recent article described girdles for men, although one "liberated" man commented that he will only wear his girdle on a first date to make a good initial impression.[20] And an advertisement for a men's gym purposely feeds into male body apprehension by warning, "No pecs? No sex!"

Scales

The counterpart of the mirror is the scale, another tool used by emotional eaters to torment themselves. While the mirror is used to critically evaluate body image dissatisfaction, the scale is used to negatively evaluate weight dissatisfaction. In one of her famous cartoons, Cathy Guisewite draws her popular character, Cathy, at home sick in bed. Cathy dejectedly intones, "I'm too sick to work. I'm too sick to read. I'm too sick to watch TV. I'm too sick to move. And yet I have the energy to leap on the scale every 15 minutes to see if I'm losing weight." She concludes morosely, "We always find the strength to do the one thing that will make us feel worse."[21]

Scales are the most popular way to determine weight loss, but they are not a precise measurement. Body weight fluctuates many times throughout the day due to different variables:

- The amount of liquid you drink.
- The size of your meals.
- The amount of salt and carbohydrates you eat which can temporarily retain water.
- Dehydration from exercise.
- Varying hormone cycles.

A scale measures the sum of your *total* body weight which also includes bone, muscle, fat, and water. And different scales yield different results!

Cynthia had an unusual relationship with the scale. She would get dressed for work—shoes and all—and get on the scale to weigh herself. She would then get completely undressed and weigh herself again in order to "prove" she had achieved some weight loss!

How often do I hear a client describe how she nudges her scale around the room, jumping on and off in the hope of finding the exact place on the floor that will reveal the lowest number. And some people do this "exercise" multiple times a day!

Interpreting Body Image Dissatisfaction

Body image self-hatred is an *emotional* problem in which we project inner conflicts of guilt, shame, sexuality, shyness, anger, and grief onto our physical appearance. Sometimes we hyper-focus on our bodies as a way to divert ourselves from a deep inner anxiety about something else that is really bothering us.

Toby had just come back from a luxury cruise in the Caribbean where she experienced overwhelming negative body "voices" in every port of call, "I'm fat. I'm ugly. I hate myself." In her therapy, Toby came to understand that her self-hatred during the cruise was actually more related to guilt about leaving her children behind while she chose to go off alone with her husband, her very first vacation without the children. Uneasy about choosing time off from being a mother ("My parents always took us kids with them on vacations") plus choosing pleasure with her husband, Toby latched on to attacking her appearance as punishment for the "crime" of enjoying her freedom.

Elizabeth, a 15-year-old bulimic girl, also targeted her body as a way to cope with anxiety. Elizabeth came to my office one day in a panic, pointing to the culprit causing her distress: a small pimple on her nose. She cried, felt unattractive, and worried that her date, Mike, would find her ugly. Objectively speaking, the pimple was not glaring. However, Elizabeth had taken all her nervousness about her date with Mike and deflected it onto the pimple.

Danny, who had struggled with anorexia and bulimia, described his own brand of body hatred. In preparation for his wedding day, he began working out feverishly. He worried that people at the wedding would secretly laugh at him for what he perceived as his protruding stomach. Through his therapy, Danny came to realize that his worry about having a protruding tummy meant that he was "like a girl" and not masculine enough. He then disclosed that he worried sometimes about whether he could be gay.

Toby's weight, Elizabeth's pimple, and Danny's stomach illustrate how we can displace our internal anxieties onto our body image. We turn our aggression against ourselves and recruit our bodies as the vehicle to express our worries.

Healing a Negative Body Image

> To me, what's sexy is when you *look like* you're having a good time.
> —Kate Upton

Many girls and women try to *look like* they feel sexy. They dress provocatively and carry themselves seductively. One girl wore pants to her therapy session with the word "juicy" scrolled in rhinestones on her backside. Another girl came to her session in four-inch stilettos, and a girl I saw on the street sported a tee shirt, "Horny for Life."

But, in fact, if you are happy in your body, you don't need to turn it into a billboard advertising your wares. It's as if these girls are trying to "look like" they feel good about themselves, as model and actress Kate Upton described above. Authentic good body image comes from inner self-satisfaction.

Because the pain of body image dissatisfaction is *emotional*, we can improve our body image through *psychological* change. Making peace with body image distress and enhancing our self acceptance involves a three-prong approach:

Awareness + Action = Acceptance

Awareness. The first step is to become aware of the physical and emotional sensations in your body and to become alert to the triggers that make you feel bad about your appearance. Are their certain people, places, or situations that most cause you unhappiness about how you look? Is it going to the gym and comparing yourself to other people there? Going out on a date? Are you triggered by clothes shopping? Visiting certain family members? Being intimate with a partner?

Practice cultivating a heightened awareness of your body's needs. Are you hungry? Tired? Cold? Sleepy?

As a young girl, Arlene was scolded by her father for being too fat. He instructed her to hold in her stomach at all times so it wouldn't stick out. Her obedience to his words, plus her own conviction that her stomach must be sucked in, persisted into her adult life. Only when she had expelled some anger to her father for his attempt to control her body was she ready to release her stomach. "I was literally waiting to exhale all my life," she said. "What's really sad is I wasn't fully aware that holding in my stomach had become so automatic." Arlene had internalized her father's rejecting message to such a degree that it continued to suffocate her many years after his death. Expelling his message was a process over time. For Arlene, exhaling involved becoming aware of the hidden rage that had caused her to unwittingly stifle herself. As she reflected on her deep need to please her father even beyond the grave, sadness and tears came welling to the surface. His spell on her was broken.

Phyllis, an obese binge eater, described how her shame about her fat body inhibited her from going to the bathroom at work. "I feel embarrassed that everyone must think about how much I eat to have gotten this fat. To then lumber off to the bathroom makes me uncomfortable that all eyes are on me, so I hold it in all day. People see I evidently can't control my eating, but at least I can control my peeing. It's too shameful to show the world I have two body needs." In her therapy, we worked on her interpretation that fat means you don't deserve to have needs and you don't deserve to take care of yourself. The day Phyllis finally felt deserving to have two needs at work and went to the bathroom caused us both to break into spontaneous applause. She replaced some of her self-consciousness with self-care.

Listen respectfully and with curiosity to whatever your body may communicate. Analyze why you may not have felt entitled to respond. And then respond. Then continue to observe if you have any further resistance or shame to taking care of your body's needs.

Action. The second step is to couple your awareness of these personal trigger points with a plan of action. When we stop, look, and listen to our self-defeating thoughts and behaviors, we can begin to intervene in the negative ways we feel about our appearance. [22]

Pay attention to your private self talk and correct your distortions. Franny thought, "Carmen got that promotion at work because she's prettier and thinner than me." Or Gary believed, "Jack got to date Pam because he has a much better physique than me and he's not losing his hair like I am."

We try to repeatedly intervene in our private self talk with healing, compassionate messages. Franny needs to reframe her thinking: "I feel angry and hurt that Carmen got that promotion. My usual tendency is to blame my looks for all my disappointments in life. What can I do now to support myself emotionally instead? Maybe I should speak with my boss about what his expectations are for me in the coming months."

Gary also needed to reframe his conclusion: "Who really knows why Pam went out with Jack? Maybe because he got up the courage to ask her out while I pick on myself and assume the whole world is as negative about my appearance as I am. My thinning hair is not my only characteristic. Let me think, instead, of the positive reasons a girl would want to go out with me."

What is your investment in holding onto a negative body image? How does it help you or keep you safe? *What would be uncomfortable or dangerous about accepting your body just as it is?*

Acceptance. You do not have to be perfect to accept the body you have. They key is to call a truce with the adversarial relationship you have with your body and work on appreciating the wondrous ways it does show up for you every day without your even having to ask. The titles of Brene Brown's *The Gifts of Imperfection* and the autobiography of Nobel Prize-winning scientist Rita Levi-Montalcini, *In Praise of Imperfection,* beautifully convey the wonderful notion that perhaps the things that make you imperfect, quirky, and unique are *not* to be tamed but, instead, embraced. Pursue pleasure that is uniquely you. Claim the individual idiosyncracies that best express a positive relationship to your body and yourself. Perhaps imperfection is the new perfection!

Andy was married with children but still liked to suck his thumb to help him fall asleep. He was ashamed and hid it from his wife by overeating instead at night. Eventually, working through his shame, he was able to claim his nighttime need for his thumb. Rochelle, a bulimic woman, loved to curl up and watch television at night with her stuffed bear, Morris, and gently pull on his fur. Even though she lived alone, she was embarrassed by the babyishness of her self-soothing ritual. When I pointed out that cuddling Morris was far healthier than standing over the toilet throwing up at night, Rochelle began to feel less critical and began accepting her personal way of comforting herself.

I recommend so frequently to my patients that they discover ways of "non-food nurturing" that one of my eating disorder groups decided to begin each group discussing their "NFNs" from the week. They coined the term NFNs to remind them of the legitimacy of looking for comfort and soothing in all sorts of ways beyond emotional eating.

Decoding one's fear of fat and body hatred is the first step towards resolving emotional eating. Once we identify what we need and feel, we can then determine how we are going to express those needs directly, without recruiting our bodies to do it for us. The more we can cultivate a deep responsiveness to our needs and the more we can cultivate a rich vocabulary to express our inner emotional selves, the less likely we will speak the language of fat and pain. As we open up the spirit of inquiry into our relationship with food, we continue our progress on the journey of declaring peace with emotional eating.

Food for Thought: Evaluating Your Body Image

If you truly lived in your body, you'd be home now.
                                        —Anonymous

One of the challenges in resolving a negative body image issue is to decode what our obsession is telling us about our inner feelings. Why do we need to magnify our faults so there is no room for enjoying our bodies? What inner emotions are we avoiding and displacing onto our bodies?

How do you evaluate *your* body image:

- How do you view yourself in the mirror each morning? With a benevolent "Hi, good morning" or a scrutiny and critique of what's wrong with your face and body today?
- Do you avoid social situations because you feel too fat?
- Do you avoid mirrors? Or do you peer at yourself with some unrelenting negative judgment?
- Is there a part (or parts) of your body that you hate?
- Have you ever tried to alter your body through chronic dieting, compulsive exercise, starving, laxatives, diuretics, or vomiting?
- Does the idea of wearing a bathing suit make you feel ashamed?
- Do you weigh yourself frequently (more than once a week)?
- What is the "magic number" you would like to weigh? How would your life be improved at that number? Did you ever weigh that number? For how long? Was your life indeed better then?
- Do you often compare your appearance unfavorably with others?
- Have you experienced hurtful episodes of being teased by family or friends while you were growing up?
- Have you ever experienced physical or sexual abuse?

- Do you feel your life would be happier if you had a different body?
- Are you obsessed by a fear of fat? How long have you felt this way?
- Did these obsessions arise in response to separation, guilt, anger, sexuality?
- What might your fat phobia be distracting you from in your current life?
- If your fat (real or imagined) had a voice, to whom would it speak and what would it say?
- What in your history has made it hard for you to claim your needs directly?

Decoding our fear of fat will help us release the energy and power to unfold our most genuine selves—needy and strong, vulnerable and independent, humorous and serious, and all the colors in between!

Spain and France: Food-Friendly and Fabulous

When I was 20 years old, I went to study in Sevilla, Spain for a year. During the year I saw only one plump person—me! I was astonished at the relationship the Spanish had with food: I would venture to say it was rapture! After a small breakfast, the Sevillanos would go off to school or work, and later head home for a delightfully large lunch and a siesta. That the town was small enough that you could walk or hop a mini-bus and arrive home shortly furthered the custom of the big meal and the siesta. Stores would shut down for the two- to three-hour lunch break, clearly demonstrating the value placed on enjoying one's meal, taking a nap, taking care of oneself, and not being a workaholic.

After work, the eating and drinking promenade began in earnest. People would stroll the streets (lots of good, fun, natural exercise) stopping at different taverns for a glass of sherry and tapas—delicious little morsels of appetizers. Some bars were famous for their cheeses.

Some were famous for seafood. Some for ham. You would sample them and move on to the next bar and the next delicacy. Great fervent discussions would ensue as to whether the pig that produced the ham had fed upon wild acorns, which was considered the premium choice. Great discussions would ensue about the wine harvest, the olive oil, the aging and merits of the various goat, sheep, cow cheeses. Tapeando was a nightly part of life, a time to greet people, to socialize, and often dance flamenco and sevillanas in the bars. Everyone from toddlers to the elderly would be swirling on the dance floor. Generations mingled happily.

Then it was time to go home for a light supper and to bed. Mañana the cycle begins again. Food and life were to be relished.

Forty years later, during a visit to Paris, I was once again surprised to discover not one overweight French person. I grew curious. Despite the restaurants overflowing with French patrons into the late hours of the night, huge bottles of wine on every table, gorgeous pastry shops with colorful tarts and cakes, cheese stores with rich and aromatic wheels and wedges, bakeries with fresh and fragrant baguettes and croissants, no one seemed to be struggling with their eating or weight. What was going on here? Could we learn anything from them? I decided to investigate.

My "scientific" studies revealed:

The French tend not to eat fake foods. I saw no artificial sweeteners, frozen dinners, pretend ice cream, sugar-free cookies, imitation butter, or fat-free cheese. Nor did I see any fast food stores except for a handful of intrusive McDonalds.

The French enjoy a vibrant café life. Rather than taking out paper cups of coffee with soggy Danish and rushing off to work, the French seem to carve out time to sit and delight in a beautiful, frothy café au lait and a croissant or a jewel of a fruit tart.

The French seem to honor mealtime rituals and do not eat standing up, on the run, or in front of the television.

The French partake of wine as a daily pleasure and do not relegate it to special occasions, as we often do. They allow themselves the enjoyment of wine with both lunch and dinner, sipping it slowly. It is an integral part of life.

And let's not forgot who invented champagne! Champagne is on every French menu; you can order it by the glass. As Winston Churchill once rhapsodized, "Champagne imparts a feeling of exhilaration, the imagination is agreeably stirred, the wits become more nimble." For the French, imbibing champagne is just business as usual.

The beautiful presentation of food makes you want to slow down and delight in your meal. Colorful fruits and vegetables artfully decorate one's plate, adding to the sensuous gratification of the meal. The visual appeal becomes part of the culinary satisfaction.

Parisians have small kitchens and need to go marketing almost every day. Shopping at the butcher, baker, or fruit and vegetable market becomes a friendly, social visit and an opportunity to pick and choose the freshest produce.

Portions are moderate. There are no supersize soft drinks, mile-high pies, steaks overhanging the plate.

And foods are flavorful, with a great emphasis on preparing what is in season and on subtle seasonings. A charming custom in many restaurants is the presentation at the beginning of the meal of an amuse-bouche. Literally meaning, "to amuse the mouth," these little appetizers are miniature works of art, with layers and layers of flavor. As you tenderly bite into these tiny morsels, the blend of flavors is surprising, exotic, and very satisfying.

Someone once said, "The amuse-bouche is the best way for a great chef to express his big ideas in small bites!" Examples of the creativity of the amuse-bouche may include tuna cubes dabbed with ginger-apricot aioli; corn soup with coconut milk; mixed greens, gorgonzola, and candied pecans; fresh pear and roasted sliver of lamb chop with orange, garlic, and rosemary pesto rub. So rather than gulping down your meal distractedly, as we Americans often do, you find yourself savoring and relishing it slowly.

Back home, I decided to read the 1995 bestseller, *French Women Don't Get Fat: The Secret of Eating for Pleasure*, by Mireille Guiliano. When I noted one chapter devoted to chocolate and another devoted to champagne, I realized this was quite different from any other weight-loss book in the United States!

Ms. Guiliano, CEO of Veuve Clicquot, describes how French women do not feel guilt or deprivation in their relationship with food. They do not diet but focus, instead, on the pleasures of food, emphasizing freshness, variety, balance, and always enjoyment. The author highlights our need for a variety of foods to genuinely satisfy ourselves. This recommendation reminded me sadly of an overweight girl who came to therapy, unable to lose weight. For one full year she had been eating nothing but tuna sandwiches every single day for lunch. She kept "falling off the wagon" with her diet and couldn't figure out why. As Guiliano says, "Deprivation is the mother of failure."

According to Guiliano, *heightened* enjoyment of eating is the key to staying in balance with food. She states, "French women take pleasure in . . . eating well, by emphasizing quality over quantity, while Americans typically see it as a conflict and obsess over it." She adds, "When you learn to replace junk with goodies that truly satisfy, you will learn that there can be an almost ecstatic enjoyment in a single piece of fine dark chocolate that a dozen Snickers bars can never give you."

Guiliano encourages Americans with a typical French expression, *"Vivre de pain, d'amour et d'eau fraiche,"* or live on bread, love, and fresh water![23]

But lest we feel too envious of the slender French—they smoke. And smoke. And smoke. And perhaps this is an unmentionable insidious habit that helps them to remain slim.

Also, the French are missing something else that makes our lives irresistible: They do not have real New York bagels. Jennifer, who worked as a waitress in Paris at a café with Jewish owners observed, "The French were always pointing to the menu and asking, '*Quest-ce que c'est un bagel?*' " or "What is a bagel?" which they pronounced *baaah-jell.*

So the French may be slim, but at least we Americans know what we're having for Sunday brunch: "A poppy seed bagel with a schmear, *s'il vous plait!*"[24]

1   Gayle King, editor of *Oprah* magazine: "I don't leave home without my Spanx. Normally I wear a large, but for an evening event, I'll squeeze into a medium. But when desperate times call for desperate measures, I'll wear *two* pairs in a large. I'm not saying it's comfortable, but it's effective! *Oprah,* October, 2012, 153.

2   Linda Lee, "Bridal Hunger Games: Losing Weight in Time for the Wedding," *New York Times*, April 15, 2012.

3   The 2012 International Conference on Eating Disorders included speakers from England, Canada, France, Switzerland, Sweden, Norway, Finland, Denmark, Spain, Brazil, Germany, Italy, Australia, and Belgium.
The television program "The Biggest Loser" has now been produced in 25 countries and shown in 90! In the Indian version, contestants do Bollywood-inspired dances to get in shape. In the Middle East edition, women must cover themselves during weigh-ins.

4   In the charming novels about a beloved African obese woman detective from Botswana, Madame Ramotswe refers proudly to her heavy body as "traditionally built." Her enjoyment of her large curves speaks of a comfort in her own skin that many African American women no longer feel. Alexander McCall Smith, *Tears of the Giraffe* (Anchor Books, 2000), 121.

5   Denise Brody "Blacks Join the Eating-Disorder Mainstream," *New York Times*, September 20, 2005.

6   On the other hand, Afghan women are now electing to undergo surgery to make their noses *bigger* to conform to the Pashtun ideal of beauty. Nose enlargement is the most popular procedure in western Kabul. The bigger the nose, the prettier it is considered. Nose reconstruction surgery requires harvesting material from the rib cage.

Nicola Smith, "Afghan Brides in Rush for Big Noses," *The Sunday Times*, October 7, 2012; http://www.thesundaytimes.co.uk/sto/news/world_news/Afghanistan/article1142042.ece.

7   Retouching grade school pictures is gaining in popularity: http://www.thedailybeast.com/newsweek/2008/02/16/say-cheese-and-now-say-airbrush.html

8   Chris Rock portrays the struggle of black women in their relationship to their hair in the 2009 movie *Good Hair*. In Spanish, good hair *(pelo bueno)* refers to being born with straight hair like white women, while bad hair *(pelo malo)* means nappy and kinky and unattractive.

9   Erica Goode, "Study Finds TV Alters Fiji Girls' View of Body," *New York Times*, May 20, 1999. Anne E. Becker, "Television, Disordered Eating, and Young Women in Fiji: Negotiating Body Image and Identity During Rapid Social Change," *Culture, Medicine and Psychiatry*, December 2004, 533–559.

10   This web site discusses the gruesome surgery of leg lengthening among the Chinese: http://indianapublicmedia.org/amomentofscience/a-painful-way-to-grow-taller/. It was finally banned in 2006: http://www.chinadaily.com.cn/china/2006-11/05/content_724833.htm.
   This web site chronicles the history of women's foot binding, which continued throughout the Chinese countryside as late as the 1950s: http://middlekingdomlife.com/guide/understanding-chinese-women.htm
   Another body part to be under scrutiny in China: A Chinese beauty contest requires the women to have nipples spaced at least 7.8 inches apart to be eligible. *Huffington Post*, "Perfectly Spaced Nipples Required in Chinese College Beauty Contest," September 7, 2012; http://www.huffingtonpost.com/2012/09/07/perfectly-spaced-nipples-chinese-beauty-contest_n_1865298.html
   A shoe catalogue arrived in my mailbox advertising Crescent shoes that are "sleek and foot-slimming." Now even our feet need to appear skinny!

11   Cathy Jenkins, "Many Young African Girls Want Lighter Skin," BBC News, January 12, 2001; http://news.bbc.co.uk/2/hi/africa/1114088.stm.
   The black singer Beyoncé has been accused of permitting "whitewashing" of her skin color to make it appear lighter for the promotional ads for her albums, as well as being airbrushed a lighter shade for a cosmetic ad. Julee Wilson, "Beyoncé Accused of Skin Lightening in New Album Promo Ad," *Huffington Post*, January 17, 2012. http://www.huffingtonpost.com/2012/01/17/beyonce-skin-ligthening-ad_n_1210377.html.

12   Obesity in Mauritania, which is most often achieved through forced feeding, has long been the ideal of beauty. It is an attempt to show off a family's wealth in a land repeatedly wracked by drought. Rukmini Callimachi, "New Views in Desert Culture on Fat Women," *Huffington Post,* April 16, 2007; http://www.huffingtonpost.com/huff-wires/20070416/mauritania-loving-fat/.

13   Media pressure has begun to call attention to the danger of fashion's stick-thin models (also called "tits on sticks"): Judith Warner, "Fashion Models and Role Models," *New York Times,* September 21, 2006; http://opinionator.blogs.nytimes.com/2006/09/21/taking-a-stand-against-stick-thin-models/. Eric Wilson, "When Is Thin Too Thin?" *New York Times,* September 21, 2006; http://query.nytimes.com/gst/fullpage.html?res=9D04EFDF1131F932A1575AC0A9609C8B63.   Kimberly Conniff Taber, "With Model's Death, Eating Disorders Are Again in Spotlight," *New York Times,* November 20, 2006; http://www.nytimes.com/2006/11/20/world/americas/20iht-models.3604439.html?_r=0. Guy Trebay, "Fashion Diary; Looking Beyond the Runway for Answers on Underweight Models," *New York Times,* February 6, 2007; http://query.nytimes.com/gst/fullpage.html?res=9E02EFDA133FF935A-35751C0A9619C8B63. Diaa Hadid and Daniella Cheslow, "New Israeli Law Bans Underweight Models in Ads, Undisclosed Airbrushing," *Huffington Post,* March 20, 2012;   http://www.huffingtonpost.com/2012/03/20/israel-bans-underweight-models_n_1366435.html.

14   Marlene Boskind-White and William White, Jr., *Bulimia/Anorexia: The Binge-Purge Cycle and Self Starvation* (W.W. Norton, 2001) 51.

15   D.M. Garner and P.E. Garfinkel, eds., *Handbook of Psychotherapy for Anorexia Nervosa and Bulimia* (Guilford Press, 1985), 6.

16   Diane Levin, Ph.D. and Jean Kilbourne, Ed.D., *So Sexy So Soon: The New Sexualized Childhood and What Parents Can Do to Protect Their Kids* (Ballantine Books, 2009).

17   The psychoanalyst D.W. Winnicott suggested that our first experience with a mirror is gazing into our mother's face. If her face is generally cold and unresponsive, then when we look into a mirror in the future, we may feel judgmental and critical of ourselves. If our mother looks at us with pleasure and affection, we have a much easier relationship with the future mirrors in our life. D.W. Winnicott, *Playing and Reality* (Routledge Classics, 1999), 111–114.

18   Advertisements often attempt to stir up negative feelings about our bodies. The scene is a beautiful, luscious tropical beach with two beckoning lounge chairs overlooking the sea and the ominous words, "You don't even want to go there . . . before you come to our office for noninvasive body contouring."

19   This article explores the hidden dangers of many seemingly benign fashions and body modification trends: Johannah Cornblatt, "Fashionably Dangerous," *Daily Beast*, July 19, 2010; http://www.thedailybeast.com/newsweek/2010/07/19/fashionably-dangerous.all.html.

This article demonstrates the dramatic airbrushing of famous models to slenderize them: Jessica Bennett, "Unattainable Beauty," *Daily Beast*, May 21, 2010; http://www.thedailybeast.com/newsweek/features/2010/unattainable-beauty.html.

The "Barbie" is the latest vaginal reconstruction surgery; it cuts away the inner labia to "improve" the appearance of the vagina: Katie J.M. Baker, "Unhappy with Your Gross Vagina? Why Not Try 'The Barbie'?" *Jezebel*, January 18, 2013; http://jezebel.com/5977025/unhappy-with-your-gross-vagina-why-not-try-the-barbie?tag=plastic-surgery.

Cindy Adams, gossip columnist for the *New York Post*, loves to spoof the body modifications of Hollywood actresses: "Hollywood's whole world is temporary. Sculpted bodies, eyes that never squint, mouths that can barely pucker. Teeth like Chiclets. Lashes like pine needles. Brows done by Picasso, fake nails, fake breasts, fake colored irises. Breaking into a smile would give the face seven years of bad luck. Hollywood—where everybody is somebody—until they become nobody." *New York Post*, March 1, 2013.

20   Neely Tucker, "Girdles for Men? Beer-bellied Guys Are Taking a Cue from the Ladies," *Washington Post*, August 19, 2010.

21   Cathy Guisewite, *Wake Me Up When I'm a Size 5* (Andrews and McMeel, 1985).

22   The *Huffington Post* reports a new trend: women who are going on "mirror fasts" and practicing "mirror abstinence." One woman took down her bathroom mirror, replacing it with a sign that said, "You look fine!" *Huffington Post*, May 2, 2013; www.huffingtonpost.com/2013/05/02/you-look-fine-how-we-wish-women-saw-themselves-photo_n_3199567.html?icid=maing-grid10%7Chtmlws-main-bb%7C-dl21%7Csec1_lnk1%26pLid%3D307788.

23   Mireille Guiliano, *French Women Don't Get Fat: The Secret of Eating for Pleasure* (Random House, 1995). However, the French are getting fatter: A 2005 survey showed 11.3 percent of the French are obese and nearly 40 percent overweight, compared with more than 50 percent overweight in Britain and the United States. Obesity has been rising 5 percent annually since 1997. Elisabeth Rosenthal, "Even the French Are Fighting Obesity," *New York Times*, May 4, 2005; http://www.nytimes.com/2005/05/03/world/europe/03iht-obese.html.

24 The Italians also deserve to be mentioned as a culture that loves their food. Sophia Loren is quoted as saying: "Everything you see, I owe to spaghetti." Although I'm not completely sure what she meant, it does sound like a wonderful tribute to Italian food. Food resonates deeply in Italy, where even the slimmest take time for proper lunches, eating several courses without conflict. There are 350 different kinds of Italian pasta, in a variety of exuberant shapes from ribbons to rods, shells, tubes, and twists. A visit to Venice revealed many glorious colors of pasta as well: green, purple, orange, black, and red. What a celebration!

5. Childhood Attachments and Eating Disorders

To celebrate springtime, a Brooklyn company decorates their large showcase window with trees and flowers with little baby chicks and eggs nestled in the grass. People love watching the antics of the fuzzy yellow babies exploring their new terrain, playing with one another, and pecking for food.

For me, the thrill is watching the chicks hatch. A little beak pokes through the egg—its first foray into the world. Then the pecking quickens, breaking through more shell. And then the baby bird takes a rest. Chicks in various stages of hatching lay on the grass with beaks and heads and fluffy bodies emerging from their shells all at their own pace. Some of the babies are vigorous, others are laid back. Some are eager to see the world, others are reminiscent of the cartoon where the baby bird peers out of his egg, doesn't like what he sees, and pulls the shell back over his head. Finally, within a few days, all are hatched and ready to meet life.

In discussing this annual chick hatching experience with one of my patients, Clare revealed, "I also like watching the eggs hatching in the store window. But then I anxiously project ahead to when the chicks become chickens and will be discarded in some unloving way. So if I were one of those chicks, I would be an anxious chick, dreading the future when I would be unloved and uncared for." Clare's reaction shows so clearly how much we bring our own history and sensitivities to interpreting life around us.

When we are born, we latch onto our parents and then, in time, through our ongoing relationship with them, we begin to *emotionally* hatch and develop, continuing to evolve into our unique selves throughout the rest of our lives.

Early childhood experiences clearly influence and set the stage for our future emotional growth. Most people believe that eating disorders just emerge out of the blue in someone's life. Nikki turns age 15 and becomes anorexic. Richard becomes bulimic at 17. Heather starts compulsive bingeing when she's 23. The truth is the seeds of anorexia, bulimia, or compulsive overeating are planted long before the actual symptoms take hold.

Attachment theory helps us understand how early life experiences contribute to a person's affliction with emotional eating disorders.

What is Attachment Theory?

I am at Jones Beach in the late afternoon. The lifeguards have gone home and people are packing up. A young couple arrives on the beach with their three-year-old son in tow. Eager to play by themselves in the ocean, they decide to hoist the child to the top of the lifeguard's chair, way high up. The father climbs up the side of the chair, deposits his son, and the couple can now have fun in the water, temporarily free of him. Terrified, the boy begins to shriek and cry. His parents are oblivious to his pleas as they jump into the waves and don't look back. Soon the boy becomes frozen and sits immobile, desperately hoping for his parents to come rescue him.

What does this little boy learn about life from this encounter with his parents? One might say, "Well, just one scary experience probably never hurt anyone." On the other hand, this experience may be emblematic of how they deal with him regularly—an ongoing pattern of disregarding him emotionally. And, if this is the case, the child is learning that his parents, and by extension others, cannot be trusted to care for him or to help him when he is in pain. He learns he is alone in the world with his fears and his fury and he is powerless.

We cannot predict this child's future, of course, but here is one imagined scenario: I picture him becoming a school bully, picking on smaller children to make himself feel more confident. Maybe later he will become a drug user to quell his pain and rage. Later, perhaps, an abusive husband. A small child's trust was shattered that day at the beach. Repeated experiences of betrayal by his parents will impact him for life.

Early experiences of bonding with our mothers, fathers, siblings, and other caretakers set the foundation for our capacity to love, to trust, feel secure, confident, and self-reliant. Through a relationship with a soothing mother—her voice, her touch, her attuned responses—we are reassured that our needs are important and will be taken care of. A child gazes at his parent's face and knows if it mirrors love and pleasure for him.

Mothering does not have to be the domain of only a mother. Any ongoing caring, tender, loving, and kind person can provide mothering. So keen is the need for mothering, that one little boy in a Romanian orphanage heartbreakingly asked, "Will a mother be coming to get me?" He did not ask for "*my* mother" but "*a* mother." When you are desperate to be loved, *any* mother will do.

John Bowlby, the famed British psychiatrist and "father" of attachment theory, states that attachment is "a lasting psychological connectedness between human beings that affects us from the cradle to the grave." The love style between parent and child will color all our close relationships—from friendships to romantic relationships as adults. These patterns, learned in childhood, persist throughout our life.[1]

Most importantly, secure and loving bonding in our early childhood shapes even our developing relationship with *ourselves*. Picture the intricate process of a parent teaching us to tie our shoes. With patience and repetition, our parent demonstrates over and over again how to crisscross the laces, make loops, pull the loop through, and form a bow. And then one day, by dint of much trial and error and loving guidance, voilà! We learn how to tie our shoes. Discovering how to respond to our own emotions is a similar learning process. With patience and repetition, our parents work to understand our needs and distress, identify what may make us feel better, and try to comfort us. By dint of this repetition—like learning to tie our shoes—we internalize the lessons of how to identify our own needs and comfort ourselves. We absorb our parents' compassionate and empathic relating and make it our own. Over time, by internalizing their caring, we eventually learn to become independent and provide emotional nourishment to our very own self. With that secure foundation, we do not need to resort to eating disorders to fortify ourselves.

As little children, we also learn ways to calm ourselves without our parent's presence: sucking our thumb, cuddling our teddy bear, having a special security "blankie"—all help bridge the gap between needing our mothers to comfort us and doing it by ourselves. As our hatching continues, we become more separate and independent from mother. This capacity to soothe one's self may be the key ingredient in preventing an eating disorder!

Ravenna, age 1½, is humming to herself in her stroller while her mother and I are engrossed in conversation. Her mother is not paying attention to her in that moment and Ravenna "entertains" herself by humming. She comforts herself by repeating the singing and humming she so often hears from her mother when they cuddle. Mother doesn't need to be tending her every minute because Ravenna can "mother" herself for a while. I bend down and say to her laughingly, "Ravenna, you are internalizing your good mother so in the future you will have resources to soothe yourself and therefore not develop an eating disorder." She looks at me curiously and starts to giggle. Her mother and I decide her first therapeutic encounter has gone very well!

The good news is that our parents do not have to understand us perfectly or respond perfectly. They just have to love us and be "good enough." If they instantly relieved all our frustrations, we would all grow up to be spoiled brats! Some disappointment is growth-promoting because we learn to tolerate frustration. Tolerating frustration and managing tension is another key ingredient in preventing an eating disorder.

But sometimes, the quality of bonding between child and parents is not "good enough," and the rhythm between parent and child is not harmonious. In the temperamental realm, some babies are mismatched with their parents—a placid baby with a vibrant, energetic parent can feel overwhelmed and want to withdraw. A lively, vivacious baby with a passive or depressed parent can feel ignored and neglected.

Complicating these unattuned attachment styles are the different feeding approaches, where parents and children may be out of sync and mismatched. Babies communicate their hunger, fullness, and the pace at which they want to be fed. Parents can "listen" and respond or, because of their own self-involvement or other limitations, override their babies' messages. From the feeding relationship, the child learns whether asking for what he needs will generally be satisfied. Again, feeding just has to be adequate and "good enough."

In the emotional realm, family problems—physical or mental illness, financial insecurity, addiction, trauma—affect parents' abilities to tend a child with consistent love and care. Sometimes parents, depleted and burdened by their own past histories of painful attachments, may not have the inner resources to adequately nourish and nurture their child.

Some needy parents may create a role reversal and recruit their child to become a parent to them. Little Ella worked earnestly to be the family clown, hoping to relieve her mother's depression by getting her to laugh. Young Max would hide his father's whisky bottles, hoping to protect his mother from his Dad's alcoholic rages. Tammy, a 30-year-old bulimic woman, was convinced as a little girl that if she kept her father's sock drawer well organized, it would stop him from gambling. And Esther, an anorexic young woman, spoke of becoming her mother's therapist after her parents' contentious divorce. "Listening to my mother's pain and anger became my 'emotional job description.' But after a while, it got so unbearable that I just wanted to block out her needing me. For self-protection, I got numb and shut down. I didn't even want to eat anymore," Esther revealed. When a child feels responsible for a parent's well-being, she learns to dismiss her own needs and to focus on trying to fix the other person's hardships instead. When our early attachment bonds are not sufficiently loving or consistent, we become uneasy about closeness and want to avoid intimacy. Insecure bonds lead to stressful tension states: anxiety, anger, worry about abandonment, an obsessive need for approval, fierce self-reliance, or compulsive care-giving.

And in these cracks, where parents and child do not mesh well or do not understand each other well, the child develops deficits in learning how to take care of himself and to respond to his own needs. The search for comfort later in life can provide fertile ground for the development of eating disorders and/or other addictions.[2]

How Does Attachment Theory Help Explain Eating Disorders?

Yolanda, age seven, and her mother go to visit her grandmother for the day. When they return home, they are shocked to discover her father has moved out without a word. His closet is empty, there is no note, and the car is gone. Yolanda is never given an explanation. Life goes on as if nothing happened. Yolanda's world is never the same. She is vigilant, on guard, frightened, angry, and confused. Yolanda is left extremely alone. A little girl's heart and trust are ruptured.

What does Yolanda learn about life from this traumatic episode?

- My father does not love me or he never would have left me.
- I must be unlovable.
- Was my whole relationship with my father fake, and I didn't even know it?
- Did all our experiences together mean nothing that he could give me up so easily?
- You can't really trust people, because you don't know what they are secretly thinking behind your back.
- Men have their own secret, hidden agendas.
- Men's needs are more important to them than their families.
- My father did not love my mother, and I never realized it.
- Did my mother contribute in any way to his abandonment? Did she know anything? Why didn't she protect me?
- Bad feelings should not be discussed. My mother did not explain anything to me.
- I was a fool to care so much about him. I will never let my guard down to let anyone get close enough to hurt me again.

I met Yolanda when she was a 33-year-old obese binge eater. She isolates, has few friends, and no ongoing successful romantic relationships.

Yolanda embarked on a long-term therapy journey with me. I loved her intelligence, her humor, her insights. She grew more confident with time, began venturing out to socialize, joined a gym, and gradually stopped resorting to bingeing as her automatic default setting for loneliness. At one point, Yolanda tentatively began to date and spontaneously asked me, "Do you ever worry that your husband will cheat on you or leave you?"

Clearly, I understood how Yolanda's own history prompted her question. I responded, "Given what happened with your father and your worries about whether men can be trusted, it's understandable you would wonder how I—or any woman—could trust and depend on a man. You have made the assumption that your father abandoning the family meant you were unlovable. His leaving had *nothing* to do with your lovability. It was his own inner instability. I believe when you reclaim the belief in what a great young woman you are, you will choose a man who would not want to risk losing you! Although there are no absolute guarantees in this world, the man you eventually choose will have just as much at stake in the relationship, and the two of you will form a mutual bond of trust. I really want you to experience that for yourself!"

When Early Attachments Fail to Nourish

Eating disorders are attachment disorders. People with an eating disorder have higher levels of attachment insecurity which causes them difficulty in managing their feelings and emotions. When early attachments fail to nourish, addiction to food or substances becomes an attempt to repair the hurt self—to offer comfort, consolation, and to fill up the vacuum within. Substances, like food, "take the edge off" and are easier to control than the uncertainty of human contact. Yolanda, like many others, learned that trusting food is safer than trusting people.

Those who have not experienced ongoing caring relationships will search outside themselves for an alternate form of safe haven. Food—starving, bingeing, purging, obsessive dieting—can become such a consuming passion. But searching for a refuge in the pseudo-security of emotional eating ultimately fails because comfort, intimacy, and love cannot be found through emotional eating.

A news story in 2012 profiled a woman with 1,200 pairs of shoes worth one million dollars.[3] She acknowledged she could not tame her compulsion to buy shoes, which she felt was due to "a lack of emotion and love" in her life. Evidently, she could not extract sufficient nourishment and satisfaction from human relationships, so she became hostage to accumulating shoes instead. She searched for something "out there" to substitute for what was missing "in here." She became attached to a sole mate, not a soul mate!

Attachment theory helps us better understand the lure of emotional eating. If a person has not developed sufficient internal resources to draw upon in times of stress, then bingeing, purging, and starving will seem like a helpful method to alleviate distress. And because insecure attachments early in life leave people wounded and mistrustful, they are not likely to turn to others for emotional support. This explains, in part, the prevalence of relapse in eating disorders. If the inner core self has not been strengthened through therapy, support groups, or a spiritual program, the person eventually falls back to emotional eating.

Psychotherapy can help a person understand and move beyond insecure attachment patterns of the past and can also restore a person's capacity for intimacy and self-care. Isolation with pastry needs to be replaced by intimacy with people.

How Can We Repair a Damaged Attachment?

When I was two years old, my parents went on vacation to Mexico without me. They left me with my grandparents which would have been a fine idea, except I had never met these grandparents before. They lived in San Antonio, Texas. We had never met; they were strangers to me. My first memory comes from this time. I was very scared of the large, booming grandfather clock in the guest room where I slept. It seemed like a threatening monster making loud bonging noises that I couldn't understand. I managed to express my fear, and my grandfather unplugged the clock for the rest of my time there. I remember feeling comforted when he responded to my fear.

What also added to my worry about being left by my parents in San Antonio was my uncertainty over whether they were ever going to come back to get me. When I was born, my parents had a darling English sheep dog, Texie, whom I loved. Before my second birthday,

Texie died. Not knowing how to explain his death to me, my mother told me that Texie had gone to live in California. I was heartbroken that my dog would leave me without saying goodbye. I didn't know where or what California was. All I knew was that Texie was abruptly gone and not coming back. Hearing that my parents were going away to Mexico sounded suspiciously like Texie going to California forever and not coming back. I was frightened and anxious.

When my parents finally did return, my mother was extremely ill, suffering from amoebic dysentery. She was unable to fully embrace me. I was aware she had changed, but I did not understand why. As her health improved, she gave me a present—a doll she had brought me from Mexico.

I took the doll and smashed her down on the floor. I protested my mother's abandonment of me. My trust in her was broken. Absence made my heart grow *frozen*, not fonder.

My mother lifted me onto her lap and cuddled me close to her. She let me cry and stroked my hair. Never once did she berate me for being an ungrateful child for breaking the beautiful doll. She recognized the anger and hurt I was feeling and soothed me. The doll went unnoticed in the corner as my mother hugged and rocked me and reassured me of her love.[4]

In the scheme of things, the rupture in the life of this little girl was not of tragic portions. It was not about war/poverty/illness/death/natural disaster/violence. But for a two-year-old child, her parents are her whole entire world—the earth, the moon, the stars.

Did this fearful separation at age two make me more anxious later in life about the deaths and separations of people I loved? Perhaps. Did this fearful separation make me more inclined to turn to the reliable comfort of food? Perhaps. There is no way to determine a clear cause and effect. But sometimes when we hark back to our early experiences, it can provide an insight into our emotional vulnerabilities and help explain why we turn to emotional eating for consolation.

There is no life that proceeds smoothly without any ruptures and abandonments. But when a child feels abandoned or misunderstood, the ability of her parents to accept their child's protest will strengthen the attachment bond and reassures the child she is still lovable despite harboring anger to her parents. She learns anger is not so dangerous and can be expressed directly. This strengthens the child's belief that relationships can be relied on which, in turn, fosters her sense of security.

What Are the Different Attachment Styles?

The bonding between child and parent is a complex dance of emotions. The attachment style that develops ranges on a continuum from secure to insecure, with shades and nuances in between. The need for loving maternal attachment in order for a baby to feel vitalized was brought home to me in an unexpected way on a backcountry road in Virginia. A young calf stood alone in a field, dejected and morose, its head down. From far on the other side of the pasture, his mother sauntered over and started to vigorously lick him up and down. The calf became animated and began to frolic and jump around, happy and enlivened by his mother's love.

Secure Attachment

Secure babies have parents who are tuned in to their children's unspoken needs and allow their children freedom to be curious and to safely explore their surroundings. When the time is right, they strive to teach their children to put feelings into words. Secure parents provide a foundation for their children to develop intimacy and autonomy, roots and wings.

Studies show that securely attached children learn to be empathic, beginning in childhood. *As their parents have been attentive to them, so they learn to be attentive both to others and to their own selves.* Ravenna, age 18 months, watches her mother stretched out on the rug with an ice pack under her. Jenny is in pain from having hurt her back. Ravenna watches as her mother finally struggles to get off the floor and stand up. The baby extends her tiny hand to her mother, offering to help her up from the floor. After Jenny scrambles to get up, Ravenna reaches down for the ice pack and hands it to her mother to comfort her. Her seeds of empathy and connection are developing.

Nourished by their intimate relationships with others, secure people have less need for emotional eating. For the most part, they can cope with difficult feelings, find ways to self-soothe, tolerate frustration, and ask for help.

Insecure Attachments

Insecure attachments between parents and children are caused by emotional ruptures and separations. Vera was hospitalized for an extended time with polio as a young child, frightened and separated from her family. Her physical and emotional scars lasted a lifetime contributing to depression and anorexia. Seth witnessed his mother's drug overdoses throughout his young life resulting in severe anxiety and bulimia.

Clinicians and researchers have identified a strong connection between these early insecure patterns of relationships and the later development of addictions. Because those with insecure attachments have so many unmet developmental needs, they feel hungry and insatiable for love and attention, but at the same time, shamed by their neediness. They believe their hunger makes them bad. Vera and Seth experienced insecurity in their early lives, eventually abusing food as their go-to coping mechanism for depression and anxiety.

Children who are neglected or abused learn to neglect or abuse themselves and their bodies. They learn to treat themselves as they were treated. Acting out with food is an attempt to compensate for unmet emotional nourishment.[5]

Along the Attachment Continuum

Although researchers claim that secure and insecure approaches are two distinct attachment styles, I observe that most people fall on a continuum between secure and insecure. Perhaps we all have aspects within us of security and insecurity, since parents rarely raise us with only one mode of relating.

Many people describe enjoying a secure childhood, but when they hit adolescence, their parents became anxious, controlling, critical, and, at times, abusive. The emerging independence and sexuality of their child may threaten some parents. "I used to have an enjoyable relationship with my father, until I started developing," said Nina, a recovering bulimic woman. "Then he became a totally different person—monitoring me and being paranoid about who I went out with. He slapped me across the face once when he thought I was wearing a sweater that was too tight." Parents who received abusive treatment during their own teenage years often repeat the same abusive pattern with their own teenagers.

Others describe having overwhelmed parents who paid little attention to them, ignoring their needs. But as time went by, when they grew up and moved out, these parents had more emotional resources and sometimes became more devoted and loving, especially when grandchildren came along. "My parents are the greatest grandparents in the world to my kids," described Mitchell, a recovering compulsive overeater. "But growing up, my brother and I basically had to raise ourselves. Our parents worked all the time and fought all the time. There was nothing left over for us."

On the other hand, sometimes a traumatic event destabilizes even a secure family and devoted parents get ground down by the suffering. "We were a great, fun-loving family until my sister died in a car accident," Jason related. "Then we all closed down from the pain, everyone in their own world. We all developed eating disorders or drinking problems and never came out of our family depression. I'm trying to find my way back to my life and to my parents through my own personal therapy."

In other instances, when parents go through their own psychotherapy, they may grow and evolve into more loving parents and become more sensitive and attentive. They learn to better empathize with their child as their therapist empathizes with them. "Through my therapist's compassionate listening to me, I have learned to be a better mother," explained Loretta. "Mary Anne really wanted to understand everything about why I hate my body and why I abuse laxatives rather than lecturing me like everyone else does. From that experience, I learned to be more curious and more tolerant in wanting to understand my son, rather than just yelling at him all the time to behave."

Although the attachment style we are originally raised with may lay the foundation for our future relationships, people are also very adaptable and can change over time. A great deal of time elapses between infancy and adulthood, so intervening experiences also play a large role in adult attachment styles. Those who grew up with ambivalent or anxious bonding can become securely attached as adults with nurturing and loving relationships. Healthy attachments provide good medicine for the body, heart, and soul.

1   John Bowlby, *A Secure Base: Parent-Child Attachment and Healthy Human Development* (Basic Books, 1988). Even our future sexual selves are determined by these early attachments. We may develop the capacity to be loving and intimate with a partner, or sexually anorexic (avoidant and fearful of sexuality), or a sexual binger (promiscuous and hungry for touch and tension release).

2   Attachment theory does not conflict with the theory that eating disorders have strong genetic and biochemical underpinnings. Rather, it adds to our understanding that these disorders are also the result of unmet dependency and developmental needs that leave certain people wounded. Vulnerable people substitute a connection to emotional eating for a connection with people.

3   Amy DiLuna, "Meet the Woman Who Owns 1,200 Pairs of Shoes," *Today*, July 27, 2011.

4   In discussing these events with my parents many decades later, I was surprised and hurt that my father made short shrift about how leaving me behind as a two-year-old caused me such anxiety. Since he absolutely trusted I would be safe with his parents, he did not imagine I would be frightened by these strangers. I then remembered his recounting his own fearful story of emotional indifference. When he was five years old and needed to have his tonsils out, his mother sent him to the doctor with his seven-year-old sister. Although it was an outpatient procedure, it did not occur to her that her little boy would be scared of this frightening medical procedure; she did not feel moved to want to be there with him and comfort him. I thought about how he repeated with me his mother's indifference to him. The emotional legacies of a parent's childhood often get passed on to the next generation.

5   Those who have pioneered and forged new ground regarding attachment styles include: M.D.S. Ainsworth et al., *Patterns of Attachment: A Study of the Strange Situation* (Erlbaum, 1978); Philip Flores, *Addiction as an Attachment Disorder* (Jason Aronson, 2011); K.E. Grossmann, K. Grossmann, and E. Waters, eds., *Attachment from Infancy to Adulthood* (Guilford Press, 2005). C. Hazan and P.R. Shaver, "Romantic Love Conceptualized As an Attachment Process," *Journal of Personality and Social Psychology*, 1987, vol. 52(3), 511–24.

E. Hesse, "The Adult Attachment Interview: Historical and Current Perspectives," chapter 25 in J. Cassidy and P.R. Shaver, eds., *Attachment Theory, Research and Clinical Applications*, 2nd ed. (Guilford Press, 2008).

6. The Family: From Conflict to Connection

From the very first moment of our lives, a connection exists between eating and deep emotions. The vital emotions of trust, dependency, security, generosity, and the acceptability of our needs begin at birth in the feeding experience with our parents. Anna Freud coined the term "stomach love" to describe the baby's early bond to the parents who feed him. Love has its origins in the satisfying feeling of being well-nourished. Family is where we learn to love and where we learn how to be loved.

Families, Food, and Feelings

Teenage Years

People usually begin to struggle with weight, fat, and calories during their teenage years. This is a time when an adolescent's identity is still "under construction" and is accompanied by enormous fluctuations between independence and dependence. The adolescent girl's maturing body, with its natural weight gain and increased body size, may provoke apprehension that she is getting fat. In a culture that idealizes thinness, vulnerable girls often feel ashamed and self-conscious of their larger breasts and hips.

For teenage boys, this anxiety is usually not as pronounced, since they generally welcome their increase in muscle strength and are proud of growing bigger and stronger. Vulnerable boys, however, may experience this development as threatening. Fearful of leaving the cocoon of childhood, they may retreat behind an eating disorder, a time-out from growing up. Eating disorders can be so consuming that they detour the boy's energy away from the tasks of forging a more grown-up identity.[1]

If all has gone well enough between parent and child in the feeding relationship and with overall emotional attunement, the teenager will enter adolescence—the time of greatest self-image and body change—with relative ease and few self-destructive impulses.

A mother will stay connected to her daughter, not becoming envious or overly critical of this emerging young woman. A father will also stay connected to his daughter by approving of her growing up so that she, in turn, will welcome her developing body as it begins to resemble her mother's.

With his son, a father will remain supportive and noncompetitive without shaming the boy's growing independence and sexuality. A mother will not feel threatened by her son's emerging masculinity and try to keep him tied to her.

In many families, however, adolescents struggle with their parents over independence, self-expression, power, control, and sexuality. If families cannot find a way to directly discuss and negotiate these emerging issues, the unresolved tensions often get detoured into the teenager's increasing obsession with food, weight, and body size.

When adolescents do not feel well understood or lack direct channels of communication with their parents, they recruit their body to "say" what they feel.

Nadya: "I'm on a hunger strike, Mom and Dad, because you never listen to how *I* feel about your getting divorced and what *I* want. You've *never* listened to me!"

Penny: "I'm going to puke my guts up until you finally believe what Uncle Eddie did to me."

Dylan: "Food is the only thing that comforts me and gives me relief. All you parents do is drink and yell. What about me? Whoever cared about me in this family anyway?"

The crisis of a child's eating disorder can have a beneficial effect. It may serve as an impetus for families to come together to discuss and hopefully resolve long-festering misunderstandings and disconnections among *all* family members.

Fathers, Daughters, and Eating Disorders

When I was 17 years old, I went to my friend Bonnie's house to help her get ready for her high school prom. Bonnie was bedecked in a long blue gown with a bouffant hairdo and a rhinestone necklace. As we waited expectantly in the living room for her date to arrive, Bonnie's father came home from work. She sat up tall and proud, eager for her father to see how beautiful she looked.

"Hi, girls," was all he said and walked into the kitchen. Bonnie and I sat there stunned. He hadn't noticed her. He didn't see anything different. He wasn't aware of her wish to impress him and be admired. Bonnie froze.

I remember feeling upset for Bonnie when I went home that night after the boy picked her up. A few years later, Bonnie became bulimic.[2]

There is *never* one reason or one cause that triggers the development of an eating disorder. It is always complex—a mixture of emotions, physiology, temperament, cultural pressures, family dynamics. But I knew, even then, from my 17-year-old perspective, that Bonnie was deeply hurt by her father's overlooking her, and this probably was not the first time. And so many years later, when I recalled this moment of pain that Bonnie experienced, I felt instinctively that her bulimia was a silent scream of protest, rage, and anguish over feeling unseen and unappreciated in her family.

Some girls, who feel unappreciated and empty inside, often say mournfully, "Losing weight is the only thing I ever felt good at. It's the only thing my father ever noticed and praised me for." Surprisingly enough, fathers of girls with eating disorders often have their own eating issues. A father who is an exercise fanatic or a father who is a compulsive overeater may be tempted to harshly scrutinize his daughter out of anxiety that she too may develop an emotional eating problem.

Fathers often underestimate what a key role they play in fostering healthy self-esteem in their daughters. What is the ideal role of a father in his daughter's development? How can fathers help prevent eating disorders in their child?

When fathers see their daughters as a whole person—intelligent, creative, funny—and not only through the lens of physical attractiveness, then the girl comes to view herself as worthy and whole and vital.

This healthy relationship between father and daughter helps inoculate the girl from becoming prey to disordered eating and body image anxiety. By focusing on her unique personality strengths, the father diminishes the girl's tendency to define herself exclusively by her appearance and weight. Too often, the default position of teenage girls is to critically focus on their looks. To have a father who takes pleasure in his daughter's companionship and opinions is a wonderful antidote to the girl's obsessing about her body.

A dad needs to express his emotions, be a respectful listener of his daughter's feelings, and share his own feelings and life experiences when appropriate. He needs to provide safety and security with flexible, respectful boundaries.

A supportive father needs to communicate how he sees his daughter's strengths and encourage her to develop her own special identity. And a father needs to deal with a certain sense of loss as his daughter grows up and is no longer Daddy's little girl.

Fathers and daughters hopefully should have fun, enjoyable times together as well. Claudia recalls fondly how when she was young, her father taught her to swim, ride a bike, and go rock climbing. "Stuff I'd never do with my mother," Claudia added. "Dad and I might not talk about emotions and feelings like I did with my mom, but being with him was an adventure. I knew he enjoyed these excursions as much as I did. We were great buddies!

"But when I became a teenager and started getting more independent, it wasn't always so easy. Dad taught me how to drive and started yelling at me when I froze at an intersection. He yelled at me again when he took me to the airport for my first flight by myself at age 17. He picked up that I was scared, and his yelling made me more nervous.

"What helped repair our relationship was his explaining to me at a later time why he yelled at me. He said, 'When I saw you afraid while driving and afraid again at the airport, I myself became worried that you wouldn't be able to do these grown-up things alone, without the safety net of my support.' My father didn't exactly apologize for being harsh to me, but his explanation about why he lashed out made me feel close to him again. I realized it all came out of his caring for me."

My personal history with my own father contained a mixture of both tender and not so tender experiences. When I was a little girl, one of my fondest memories with my father often occurred when he came home from a long day at work. My father was a baker. He'd arrive home and sit down to read the newspaper before dinner. I would climb onto his lap. Little lumps of dough would be caught on the hairs of his arms from his day of baking. I would sit there and "groom" him—pulling off the clumps of dough. He read the paper as I cuddled against him until I would occasionally pull too hard and yank his arm hair. He would drop me off his lap with an "Ouch! That hurt." I would come squealing back to his lap, laughing and promising I would be more careful. It was great fun for me and an intimate way of being near my father.

On the other hand, one of the worst memories was the afternoon my father and I went food shopping together. He wheeled the cart and asked me to pick out which cookies I wanted. I was happy to be allowed to choose and put the chocolate chip cookies in the cart. "Do you want more?" he asked. I couldn't believe his generous offer since my mother invariably monitored every morsel of food I put in my mouth. I chose the Oreos. "How about more?" he asked. And each time he repeated the question, I delightedly added another kind of cookie to the basket. I was so happy with this abundance. When I was done, he laughed harshly and mocked me accusatorily, "Do you really think you need all these cookies? Do you really think I'm going to buy all these for you? What's the matter with you?" I was stunned, ashamed, and betrayed. I hated him for setting me up. It was not one of our more loving moments.

Fathers, like mothers, can be a mixed bag, often blending warmth and love with cruelty and humiliation. Hopefully, the good connections outweigh the hurtful ones. We learn our parents are just human, a mosaic of good and bad.

Of course, how a man treats his wife will become the child's role model for how men treat women. If a father demeans his wife, the girl will learn that she, a female, cannot expect loving treatment from men. But if a father values his wife's opinions and treats her respectfully as a partner, the girl will learn about sharing and mutuality between husband and wife. By feeling good about herself as a growing female, she will not need to retreat behind an eating disorder.

Even though women increasingly hold prominent positions in the workplace and the professions, fathers traditionally have a strong impact on their daughters' work identity. A caring father will discuss with his daughter how he handles his job, what it's like to be out in the world with bosses and coworkers, and how to manage money. As a teenager begins to explore her interests, a father can be helpful by identifying her skills and strengths and fostering her vision for the future. He may say, "You're very creative. I could see you doing something in the advertising world. I wonder if you would like that?" or "You've always been such a great writer. Would you consider going into journalism?"

A father may also offer a different energy and perspective than the mother. Because girls tend to identify with their mothers, the father's masculine contributions can help the girl become more separate from mom and develop her own unique identity. Dad can provide a wedge between mother and daughter that promotes healthy separation between them and prevents them from being too enmeshed. His unique parenting role is "other-than-mother."

Although girls yearn to have a separate relationship with their fathers, it is important that a father not convey he is choosing his daughter in place of her mother. Nor should a mother feel abandoned and resentful of their connection.

Lucia, in recovery from compulsive overeating, spoke of her guilt and anxiety about leaving her mother behind when her father took her to see Italian movies at his Italian Cultural Club, where the movies are shown without subtitles. "My father and I are bilingual, but Mama doesn't speak Italian," Lucia explained. "Going out with him felt uncomfortably like a date, like I was his second wife rather than just a father–daughter outing. But he was very insistent I learn about his culture. I wish the three of us could have done something together as a family instead."

In *Women and Their Fathers: The Sexual and Romantic Impact of the First Man in Your Life*, author Victoria Secunda illuminates many aspects of the father–daughter connection. She describes five patterns of paternal love: the doting father, the distant father, the demanding father, the seductive father, the absent father.[3] I would add the competitive and the abusive father.

From my clinical experience, I think most fathers contain a blend of many ways of relating. I look at fathering along a continuum that ranges from caring, communicative, and compassionate to critical, competitive, and controlling. Of course, the reassuring news is that no one has to be the perfect parent. A father only has to be "good enough" to help his girl cultivate healthy self-esteem and body image.

When a daughter develops an eating disorder, she cries out about her unmet desire for loving connection in her family. The disorder is her indirect way of communicating, "All is not well in my family. All is not well with me." Trisha discussed the impact of her father's monitoring the fat content of what she ate and weighing her weekly: "I was afraid of displeasing him, so I learned to sneak food behind his back to eat what I wanted. Sneaking food became a lifelong pattern until I came to therapy. I never learned to have a healthy relationship with food or my body, just a critical one."

As well as needing to play a strong role in his daughter's life, a father also needs to play an active role in her recovery from an eating disorder. In my practice, I have been heartened by the increasing number of fathers committed to participating in their daughter's therapy for eating disorders.

As fathers and daughters learn to understand each other better and express themselves directly, everyone is enriched. The girl no longer will need her eating disorder to speak for her.

Mothers, Daughters, and Eating Disorders

> A boy is a son until he takes a wife, a girl is a daughter for the rest of her life.
>
> —Irish proverb

Once upon a time, I was born to a mother who was five feet tall and weighed 85 pounds. My mother was not especially interested in food, and so she viewed my normal, healthy appetite with some anxiety. She began to scrutinize my food—watching what I ate, doling out my portions, hiding the cookies. Since I intuitively could sniff out where the cookies were hidden, I always found the secret stash. At the same time, I feared I would be found out and was ashamed of my behavior. I began to obsess about cookies, food, sneaking and not getting caught, fear of my mother, and gaining weight.

My mother believed her intention was helpful—she did not want me to get fat. But she inadvertently created such apprehension and self-consciousness in me that it interfered with my internal healthy mechanism of knowing when I was hungry and when I was full. In her over-control of me, her good intentions backfired, and I became an emotional overeater during my childhood and teenage years.

Compared to my tiny mother, I felt huge by comparison as a young teenager. After surpassing her in height and weight, my body image was shaped by my comparison to her: Big was the verdict. And Big was not good.

Although Beth, an obese girl, came for therapy for binge eating, she could not understand why everyone hassled her about her weight. Despite being short and over 200 pounds, she did not feel over-weight. I then learned Beth's mother weighed more than 400 pounds. Compared to her large mother, Beth felt normal.

Roberta's mother was clinically anorexic. Roberta, a 20-year-old girl who was slender and pretty, compared herself critically to her mom. Mom's alarmingly low weight seemed ideal to her daughter, and Roberta was despondent she could not be as thin.

A girl often evaluates her size and shape in comparison to her mother's. I was not large nor was Beth small nor was Roberta fat, and yet our mothers' weight played an integral part in our own body image perception.

Mothers' feelings about their appearance also make a strong impact on their daughters' self-esteem. Joanna related, "When I was 11, my mother was getting ready for a party. I watched her in the bathroom as she brushed her hair. Suddenly she threw the brush against the mirror, shouting at her own reflection, 'You're ugly! I hate you!' Although she was not directing her anger to me and I knew her outburst had nothing to do with my being overweight, I was traumatized by the rage she felt against herself. I am her daughter. I look like her. It made me worried that I'm ugly too." Joanna's story demonstrates how sensitive girls are to their mother's body image issues.

As girls approach adolescence, mothers and daughters *both* have to navigate a balance between closeness and distance. The girl identifies with her mother as female, on one hand, yet also needs to discover her unique, distinctive self. This fluctuating dance between staying connected to mother and yet wishing to branch out from her can be fraught with conflict. The girl's wish for separation may leave her feeling guilty and disloyal, as if she is betraying her mother by growing up. This is especially true if the mother requires ongoing companionship or validation from her daughter and feels threatened if the girl does not want to follow in her footsteps. If the daughter tries to separate, this mother may feel rejected which contributes to the girl's guilt. A teenager may seek to remedy this problem by retreating to the comfort of food through bingeing, purging, or even through starvation.

The struggles between mother and daughter often foster eating disorders because food provides a retreat from the real world. It is the cheapest, safest, legal, and most available drug on the market. Issues between mothers and daughters that may foster the development of emotional eating include:

Pressure to be sexual. Some mothers enjoy turning their little girls into miniature sex objects, dressing them in outfits more "tart" than "tot." Makeover parties for five-year-old girls, thongs for seven-year-olds, prostitute costumes for Halloween, children's beauty pageants with bouffant wigs and makeup, dolls with miniskirts and fishnet stockings, two- piece bikinis for little girls are all for sale.

Brooke Shields' mother, who allowed her daughter to play a child prostitute in the movie *Pretty Baby,* stated, "Fortunately, Brookie was at an age that she couldn't talk back."

The *New York Times* explored these phenomena in "Hot Tots, and Moms Hot to Trot." Mothers need to vigilantly filter out hypersexual images and to reject the early sexualization of their daughters as encouraged by the media. There is a strong link between the development of eating disorders and the precocious pressure to be sexy.[4]

Envy. The girl may envy the relationship between her parents as well as their sexual intimacy. She may envy her mother's established, comfortable life, and that mom is smarter, has money, and is more powerful than she is.

On the other hand, the mother may envy her daughter's youthful good looks. She may resent the girl's freedom to go out and enjoy herself and meet boys, without the brunt of adult responsibilities. She may begrudge her daughter's opportunities and options in the world that she never had.

Competition. Mothers and daughters may compete for the attention and approval of the husband/father. Although the daughter may want to be her father's favorite, she does not really want to win the competition and risk alienating her mother. Mothers and daughters may also compete for who is more attractive and slender. Some mothers have been known to act seductively with their daughters' boyfriends.

"I never felt I could measure up to my successful mother," stated Cathy, a 20-year-old bulimic girl. "She told me, 'If you turn out to be half the woman I am, you'll be lucky.' I didn't know whether to cry or scream when she said those things. I just knew I couldn't compete with her, so I gave up. And I threw up."

Amy described an ongoing competition with her mother for who was the thinnest. "We went to a coffee shop, and I noticed when I turned my back, my mother added extra cream to my coffee. I know this sounds crazy but I'm positive she wanted to give me extra calories so she could win the skinny competition between us."

Criticism. The "best" way for a mother to subtly discharge her envy and competition is to criticize her daughter's weight. This is the ultimate psychological weapon a mother can wield: "You need to lose some weight." "You're getting fat." "Even your older sister doesn't weigh as much as you." "Your father said you really should go on a diet."

Ridiculing a child never works; it sets the stage for rebellion. Melanie reported that her sister always could have ice cream, while her parents forbade her and monitored her closely so she would not gain weight. Justine described her grandmother's humiliating week-end weigh-ins in front of the whole family. Both these women became bulimic.

How do we translate the meaning of a mother's criticism of her daughter into emotional language? The mother's disapproval may be communicating:

- You are moving away from me and I want to cut you down to size to hurt you.
- You're too full of yourself. (Or, as we say in Brooklyn, "She thinks who she is.")
- I'm afraid you don't need me any longer. What will I do with my life?
- Don't grow up and leave me alone with your father.
- You're not as pretty as you think you are.
- If you're overweight, it will make me look bad to the other mothers. I need you to be prettier and skinnier than your friends, which will prove I'm a great mom.
- I hate my own body. Why should you feel better about yourself than I do?

Dawn, age 15, struggled with a severe compulsive overeating problem. She explained the connection with her mother, "My mom gives us everything materially but nothing of herself. Instead, all she does is pressure me not to eat. But, if I'm ever going to stop overeating, the decision will have to come from me. My brain and stomach don't get along just like me and my mother don't get along."

Every mother has the awesome challenge of raising a daughter who is self-confident, with good self-esteem, positive body image, healthy eating habits, a girl who has the capacity to grow emotionally, enjoy her life, and learn to accept her imperfections without beating herself up.

The best way a mother can raise a secure daughter is to provide a strong role model by demonstrating good feelings about her own body. Unfortunately, growing up in our culture, mothers do not necessarily have an easy time either with their own body image acceptance. In *Cinderella Ate My Daughter,* author Peggy Orenstein offers a critical analysis of how our culture harms little girls' self-esteem, and yet she also ruefully acknowledges her own persistent body image problems:

> Although my body and I have reached if not peace, at least a state of détente, "fat" remains how I experience anger, dissatisfaction, disappointment. I feel "fat" if I can't master a task at work. I feel "fat" if I can't please those I love. "Fat" is how I blame myself for my failures. "Fat" is how I express my anxieties. It frustrates me to consider what else I might have done with the years of mental energy I have wasted on this single, senseless issue.[5]

Mothers often think they keep their eating problems so well hidden that there is no need to discuss their issue with their children. I don't believe it. Many adults have reported in their therapy that as they were growing up, they could hear their mother throwing up in the bathroom, or raiding the kitchen in the middle of the night, or spitting out chocolate into a napkin. In the autobiography *This Mean Disease: Growing Up in the Shadow of My Mother's Anorexia,* a son describes his devastating experience as a child of watching his mother's anorexia slowly and painfully rob her of life.[6]

By being honest with her child (to the extent it is appropriate) about her own eating issues, a mother shows she is not letting shame and embarrassment get in the way of admitting her problem. This may prompt the child to share her own struggles more readily. Hopefully, it may become another way for a parent to be a role model by revealing that it is all right to release what is locked up inside, rather than keeping shameful secrets.

Still, a mother with her own eating or body image battles will naturally have a hard time setting a helpful example for her child. Virginia, grappling with a binge eating disorder, took a direct approach. She ingeniously and unapologetically advised her daughter, "I'm such a great role model to you in every way except my eating. So learn from my good points. As for my eating issues, until I get them more in control, I'd like to help you *not* follow in my footsteps!"

Virginia could not deny that her daughter observed her eating problems. When Melissa was four and her mother had gained significant weight from her bingeing, they were cuddling in bed and Melissa piped up, "Mommy, there is less room in the bed with you now!"

I have also witnessed on several occasions how three generations of women in the same family will struggle with eating disorders. I have treated women whose mothers and grandmothers had body image issues and women whose mothers and daughters had eating disorders.

In order to break this chain and not pass on a legacy of hurtful patterns of eating and body image to one's daughter, mothers should increase their own awareness of their eating, weight, and body image history.

Think back to your own girlhood, when you were the same age as your teenage daughter:

1. How did you feel about yourself at that age?
2. What messages did you get from your mother about your body?

From your father? Your friends?

3. How do you think your mother felt about her body and size? Her eating?

4. Did she complain about her weight or her size? Or was she relatively confident in being her own person?

5. Did your father criticize her?

6. Now that you are a mother, how are you similar to you own mother?

7. How are you different from her?

8. How does your daughter feel about her body?

9. *Is there anything supportive about eating and body image that you might have liked from your mother when you were growing up that you could now pass on to your daughter?*

The best gift a mother can give her daughter is to address and resolve her own struggles to become a more positive role model. That includes refraining from making negative comments about your own body or anyone else's. If you are anxious about how you look in a particular pair of jeans, ask only your husband that famous female question, "Do I look fat in this?" Ask this out of earshot of your children. Your children are taking mental notes. Model a value system that emphasizes *inner* qualities.[7]

When a mother is comfortable enough in her own skin, has sufficiently resolved whatever food/body image issues she may have, enjoys her relationship with her spouse and friends, and has fruitful work or other creative endeavors, she will be freer to take pride in her maturing daughter. A mother who has improved her own self-esteem will invariably create a happier daughter and derive much pleasure in bringing up a young woman who genuinely likes herself.

Fathers, Sons, and Eating Disorders

> My mind is never completely empty of my father.
> —Geoffrey Wolff, *The Duke of Deception:*
> *Memories of My Father*

The number of men I have treated is significantly less than the hundreds of women I have worked with. This makes it easier to study the possible common themes that males with eating disorders share. I do not claim that my experience is valid for all, but these are my observations.

All the teenage boys and men I have worked with—be they compulsive overeaters, bulimics, or anorexics—express deep and significant disappointments in their relationship with their fathers. Beginning as young boys, they craved a strong father they could admire and who would admire them. They sought a bond based on love and mutual respect. But that was not the case among the males in my practice. Some fathers were physically abusive and beat their sons, some fathers abandoned their families, some fathers were alcoholics or drug abusers, some travelled extensively for business leaving the boy bereft of his consistent presence, some fathers had problems with the law, some were politicians or wealthy businessmen who seemed to prefer their vocations over their families. Some had hidden stashes of pornographic material. Some fathers had died, many had serious relationship problems with their wives, and some were divorced and remarried, with new wives and new children.

And, even when fathers were physically present, many lacked empathy and compassion for their sons, causing their growing boy to have inner "father hunger."[8] Some fathers let their sons know they cheated with other women, eroding the boy's sense of security and belief in his father's integrity. When a dad (or mom) repeatedly hurts a child's self-esteem, that child learns to turn away from relying on his parents for emotional nurturing and relies instead on attempts to self-nurture by purging, starving, bingeing, or obsessive dieting.

In addition, many of the eating disordered men in my practice are first- or second-generation Americans whose parents or grandparents left southern Europe to escape grinding poverty or eastern Europe to flee religious persecution. Many escaped the Holocaust in Poland to come to Brazil or Mexico and then to America. Some families fled religious persecution in Hungary and went to Chile and then New York. Several families left Egypt to make a new life in Cuba, only to be forced to flee for a second time when Castro came to power.

These are traumatic disruptions. To be forced by poverty or violent persecution to leave your country, your home, your language, your family, your business for an unknown country where you do not speak the language, where you are bereft of family and community, and with no immediate way of making money was devastating and terrifying.

The legacy passed on from these fathers to their sons, my patients, was about survival, success, being strong, being a man's man. These fathers, experiencing early ruptures in their own lives, put great emphasis on being tough and making money. They gave little importance to feelings; they were intolerant of emotional weakness in their sons. The thrust of life became the security of money, not the expression of emotions. After all, who had the chance to ponder their feelings when the Nazis were exterminating your people?

Many men with eating disorders feel they have to make good on their grandparents' and parents' sacrifices and to just suck it up. Having emotions is a luxury they could not afford. To numb the father hunger they cannot express openly, many of these men turn to food as a way to fill up their inner emptiness.

One bulimic boy who needed to be hospitalized at an eating disorder rehabilitation facility was advised by his father, "Just think of it as summer camp." Such was the father's emotional disconnection from his son's fear, pain, and shame.

Many men with eating disorders coincidentally (or not) are involved in a family business. They began their early work lives with strong anxiety about whether they could measure up and make their father and/or grandfather proud. One man anxiously binged every time he tried to close a deal as he heard his father's voice (from the grave, six feet under) saying, "*I could have put this deal together better than you.*" One young man stopped eating when his father placed him in charge of an isolated outpost of the family company. Ashamed to tell his father he was afraid to be out there on his own, he became bulimic and was forced to come home.

Many eating disordered men express a range of emotions, from craving their father's respect and admiration, to anxiety about sustaining the business once the father retired or died, to guilt for wanting to compete and outstrip the father's success.

Gene, who at age 32 earned more money than his father, felt apprehensive about this achievement and wanted to protect his father from feeling inadequate. Gene developed anorexia and through his therapy realized, "Dad recently had a heart attack and I felt my business success was another attack on him. My anorexia helped me 'diminish' myself out of guilt. I didn't realize what I was doing when I stopped eating. But when Dad became the strong one again and had to help me get well, I felt less scared. We've done some father-son therapy sessions together. I learned he is not as threatened by my success as I thought. That's a relief. Now, why did I assume that in the first place?"

Grown men may still have father hunger. In the essay "Remembrances of My Father," author Charles M. Blow relates "no matter how estranged the father, no matter how deep the damage, no matter how shattered the bond, there is still time, still space, still a need for even the smallest bit of evidence of a father's love."[9]

When a father continues to live with the hurtful messages from his own childhood, he may inadvertently repeat these patterns with his son. The pressure to be macho is handed down from one generation of men to their sons to their sons' sons. As William Wordsworth wrote, "The child is father to the man." A legacy of not expressing feelings, of being a "tough hombre" who grins and bears it, is detrimental to the healthy emotional development of boys. That model values stoicism and a constricted definition of what it means to be male—a strong, silent caricature, where feelings are considered a weakness and just for sissies and girls.

Boys, beginning at a young age, are not encouraged to develop an inner emotional life. This leads them to an existence of silence, solitude, and distrust. If a boy is taught that to be manly means denying pain and tears, his inner turmoil may surface through eating disorders, alcoholism or drug abuse, failure at school, social isolation, and depression.

In *Raising Cain: Protecting the Emotional Life of Boys*, the authors state, "There is little that can move a man to tears. . . . When a grown man cries in therapy, it is almost always about his father. The man may be hated or revered, alive or dead. The story may be one of a father's absence, his painful presence, or his limitations of spirit and feeling. The word *love* rarely comes up in the stories men tell, but that is what these stories are all about. Fathers and sons are players in a tale of unrequited love—a story told in yearning, anger, sadness, and shame."[10]

Ideally, to foster a strong sense of loving and caring masculine identity in his son, the father should serve as an example of an emotionally integrated man his son can admire and want to learn from. This presupposes a father has worked through his own father hunger about his own dad. How a father communicates his feelings about his male body, eating, sexuality, work, and his relationship with his wife are key ingredients in a son's development. How a father resolves conflicts—whether he expresses his opinions thoughtfully and respects others—will provide an example for his child to follow. By teaching his son to talk through a problem and that it is OK to verbalize confusion or discomfort, a father provides a powerful coping tool—the value of expressing feelings, rather than reverting to emotional eating as a way to discharge them.

When parents recognize that boys can be needy, vulnerable, tearful, dependent, and fearful just like girls, they break the cycle of the stiff-upper-lip pattern of male development. Then boys are free to express a full range of emotions—fear, confusion, worry, tenderness, and love. When parents respect the inner emotional life of their sons, these sons flourish and cultivate self expression. No need for an eating disorder here.

Mothers, Sons, and Eating Disorders

Sugar and spice and everything nice,
That's what little girls are made of.
Slugs and snails, and puppy dog tails,
That's what little boys are made of.—Nursery rhyme

Many men in my practice had more involved relationships with their mothers than their fathers. Often, the son became the mother's confidante, silent witness to his mother's secrets with her injunction, "Don't tell your father." Often, the son was cast in the role of the daughter that Mom never had. Mother and son would go to Weight Watcher meetings together, for example, and count calories, an activity more often shared between mothers and daughters. Sometimes a mother would use her son as an emotional replacement for a distant or neglectful husband.

One mother would cry out, "Thank God you're here," when her son came to visit, as if he were the messiah saving her from her unfulfilling marriage and the boredom of her life. Another mother had an affair she instructed her son to keep secret from her husband. One mother sexually abused her son after her husband abandoned the family. Another mom would tell her son how she wished he were a girl.

For some mothers, a son can seem like an alien creature, filled with "slugs and snails and puppy dog tails." He feels so different from a familiar little daughter of "sugar and spice and everything nice." Mothers who have strife with their fathers, brothers, or husbands or a history of abuse may not feel particularly comfortable with males. They may fear the normal rambunctiousness of boys. The mother may shy away or try to shut her son down, anxious that his male energy means he is out of control.

Ingrid, a married woman with a long-term history of anorexia and bulimia as well as sexual abuse by her grandfather, was terrified to learn she was pregnant with a son. Ingrid believed her son would be born almost full-grown and would come to dominate her emotionally and sexually as her grandfather had done. As strange as it sounds, Ingrid was relieved when her son was born a tiny, little baby with a tiny, little penis.

And then there are mothers who hope their sons will become their strong protectors. As the authors of *Raising Cain* put it, "Nobody wants to think of boys as depressed or emotionally needy. We feel embarrassed or uncomfortable with the shame it will bring them, and we feel more secure with the idea that these idealized 'strong' fathers-in-training can protect us with their strength."[11] They go on to point out that in healthy development, a boy and his mother navigate a delicate balance: "As he grows, a boy must be able to leave his mother without losing her completely and return to her without losing himself. At each point, a mother must adjust her connection, providing both the emotional grounding and the emotional freedom her son needs to grow."[12]

Good mothering means not focusing exclusively on external proof of her son's value, such as grades, sports achievements, or trophies. When a boy feels loved unconditionally for just being himself, he learns externals are not as important as his inner, authentic self.

This kind of genuine bond can make the mother–son relationship wonderfully enjoyable. One young boy spent his childhood watching his mother, a professional dancer, teach ballroom classes. For years he observed as she instructed her students on rhythm, balance, and foot placement. This boy became a talented and skilled surfer, achieving rhythm, balance, and foot placement on the surfboard! Perhaps neither mother nor son made the connection that he absorbed what he learned from her and translated it into his own unique arena. Her medium was the dance floor, his, the ocean. Mothers teach sons how to play the piano, cook, drive, sing, play tennis, speak Spanish. One mother, a psychologist, often discussed human dynamics as her son was growing up; he became a renowned filmmaker exploring psychological themes in his movies. And sons, in turn, may teach mothers about computers, smartphones, and all the latest gadgetry.

A mother–son relationship that really blooms includes the mother sharing her feminine beliefs while respecting the masculine differences of her son. And she includes big doses of humor and fun. As one mother affectionately said, "I want my son to be tough and tender. Both."

Family Therapy
An adolescent's eating disorder presents a crisis for the whole family. Hopefully, the parents will seek out family therapy to unravel why their child has gotten stalled. Because an eating disorder can be a time-out from growing up, family therapy focuses on helping the youngster get unstuck and continue to grow through the developmental transitions of adolescence. In addition, family treatment can help parents negotiate their own relationship as husband and wife as well as learn to be consistent, effective parents of a teenager. A 16-year-old daughter requires quite different parenting skills, discipline, and boundaries than when she was six.

One of the fathers in my practice, Rick, loved being the soccer coach for his daughter's team. When Samantha reached 15, she no longer wanted to spend her weekends playing soccer, but Rick insisted. It had become so much a part of *his* identity that he hated giving it up! Samantha, ready to move on from the time constraints of soccer, protested, but Rick was adamant. She slowly lost interest in school, began restricting her food, and was headed down the road to becoming anorexic. Since her out-loud protest did not carry any "weight," now her body was not carrying weight.

When Rick arranged a family consultation with me, it became clear that Samantha was both furious and guilty at having to please her father. She had begun a hunger strike. Samantha knew she was depriving her father of pleasure by turning her back on the sport they had shared. Her anorexic behavior became her justification not to play, an indirect expression of anger at him. At the same time, it served as a self-punishment for hurting her dad.

Family therapy uncovered how during Rick's own youth, he had yearned for *his* father to have been as hands-on with him in sports as he was with Samantha. Family sessions also worked to strengthen the ties between Rick and his wife, Joyce, which had eroded over many years. Joyce began to reveal her anger at being left behind for all of Samantha's and Rick's soccer outings. She had never previously complained, because she also appreciated Rick's involvement with Samantha, something she had lost at age 10 when her own father died.

This family was unusual because traditionally mothers are overly close to their children and fathers are overly distant. Nevertheless, all family treatment seeks to balance the equilibrium. Family therapy illuminates the various relationship entanglements to find more gratifying ways of helping the entire family enjoy their connections more. Family therapy supports opening up communication among *all* family members so everyone can have their needs expressed and addressed more directly so all members can flourish.

Family treatment also affords siblings a chance to voice their concerns. Joel and Stella were given the floor to speak about how their sister Nicole's anorexia affected them. Joel started to fail in school and, in the therapy, he voiced his anger that Nicole, his anorexic sister, was getting all the attention. "Because she's the sick one, there is nothing left over for me. My parents act like they have only one child—Nicole—and I'm very pissed off."

Stella had the opposite reaction from her brother. Sensing how worried and overwhelmed her parents were about Nicole, Stella bent over backward to "be good." She tried to help out more around the house, retreated into herself, and became depressed with insomnia. "I'm feeling like a lost soul," she cried in the family sessions.

The parents were alarmed to learn how Joel and Stella felt; it was true that their absorption with Nicole had derailed them from being the parents of *three* children. Discussions with the five of them led to changes in how they related to one another. The parents recognized they could not let Nicole's illness erode the whole family, and they sought additional support for her. Nicole also voiced her guilt about her anorexia, which helped her siblings realize she really was sick and not just being selfish. This family was strengthened as family members listened to each other and appreciated that suffering in silence was not the solution.

Another troubled girl, Fern, benefited from family treatment. Fern described, "My father always treated my mother like dirt, belittling her all the time. I felt terrible for her, but I was also angry because she never stood up to him. I was also angry that Daddy was so belligerent, but I felt sorry he was married to such a frightened mouse like my mother. I didn't know whose side to take. It was awful. I felt so guilty. I became bulimic. Bulimia helped me push down my turmoil with my parents and gave me a way to forcefully expel a lot of rage. Thank goodness for my bulimia, because it pushed us into family therapy! In sessions I got to shout and unload tons of stuff about what was wrong with our family. It really helped us eventually iron out our family baggage. Now, after a lot of blood, sweat, and tears," laughed Fern with relief, "we don't have heavy family baggage any longer—just the usual light carry-on luggage!"

Preventing Eating Disorders: Why Childhood Matters

My cousin Rachel came to visit for the weekend with her 3½ -year-old daughter, Sophie. I was surprised Sophie had gotten fat—not just chubby, but fat—since the last time I had seen her. I wondered if this weight gain was genetic or whether her eating behavior was out of kilter. Over the weekend I tried to figure out the answer by observing mother and child.

When Sophie was playing in the garden, her mom would call out, "Come eat now. Let me give you a sandwich." Sophie, interrupted from her playing, took her mother's cue as a new fun activity and marched into the house to eat. Rachel did not consider whether Sophie was really hungry at the time. Nor did Rachel realize that if Sophie were really hungry, she would have initiated asking for food.

Throughout the weekend, Sophie would whine that she wanted something to eat, and Rachel would feed her at every occasion. Rachel never took time to find out if Sophie was genuinely hungry or just bored or tired or looking for her mother's attention. There seemed to be no structure or any kind of limitation to Sophie's constant eating demands, mostly for sweets and snacks.

We know that childhood is a crucial time for parents to help their children form lifelong patterns of healthy eating. Although eating disorders may not arise until adolescence, the seeds of eating problems are planted in the young, formative years.

Ellyn Satter, a clinical social worker and registered dietician, has researched and pioneered specific concepts to help parents feed their children nutritionally and joyfully. She states that both the parents and the children share the responsibility of healthy eating. The job of the parent is to decide *what* they feed their children, *when* they feed, and *where* they serve food. Children also share the responsibility: They get to decide *how much* of the food they want to eat and *whether or not* they choose to eat at all.[13]

Lynn, a recovering binge eater, discussed her plight, "I have four kids and always wanted to get them to eat well and give them what they want, but each one has different food preferences. Sometimes I feel like a short-order cook trying to please everyone. Then I reached my boiling point. With my therapist's encouragement, I now make one meal—whoever doesn't want to eat it doesn't have to. In trying to be a good mother, I just gave away my personal power. Now I feel so liberated and no longer a slave to my kitchen or the kids. And no one is starving to death!"

Parents need to teach their child the lessons appropriate for each stage of development. For babies, the task of the parent is to feed them on demand, when the baby indicates it wants to be fed. In the past, pediatricians recommended that parents put their child on a rigid feeding schedule. We now know that babies need to be fed when they are hungry, not according to some preordained structure that is external and not connected to the child's internal and varying needs.

When parents allow their baby to determine when to eat, how much, how fast or slow, and when to stop, the child learns that hunger or fullness is valid and respected. The baby should set the rhythm and the parents take the cues.

Often, a mother with her own history of disordered eating is uncomfortable letting her baby take the lead in the feeding. Just as the mom never learned to trust herself with food, she does not trust her baby to get it right either. Mothers have said to me, "I don't want my baby to get fat and have the same weight problems I have, so I'm going to make sure not to overfeed her. If she cries for more food, I'll just try to distract her." Others have said, "I want to get as much food into her as possible so she won't feel deprived like I did." *Both* positions—depriving or overindulging the baby—set the stage for future eating problems.

However, the beauty of feeding babies on demand is that we teach them the world is an abundant place where their needs get met. This, in turn, helps them learn to eat when they are hungry and stop when they are full. As a child matures, he learns to integrate this feeding on demand as a way to feed himself for life. The child learns that food is only about food, not an emotional stress reliever.

In my practice, I have seen an exciting outcome when mothers come for therapy for their own emotional eating problems. The topic that invariably arises is the mom does not want to pass on her eating struggles to her child. I teach parents the importance of on demand feeding for their babies, and *how that very same feeding technique can repair their own disordered eating patterns.* Through learning how to be responsive to their baby's feeding cues, many mothers learn to apply the same empathic attunement to themselves. Some women only know how to diet. As they learn to trust their baby's expression of hunger and fullness, they can also learn to trust their own bodies, feed themselves when hungry, and stop when full.

I strongly believe the following principles will help to prevent eating disorders in children:

Dieting is not the answer. Dieting is not recommended for children, even those who are overweight. Dieting lowers a person's metabolism. Research shows that dieting in children and teens not only increases the risk of obesity but also sets the stage for potentially hurtful eating disorders. Teach children to eat when they're hungry, stop when they're full. Help them increase activity levels, make better food choices, and curtail emotional eating through talking empathically about their feelings.

Be flexible. The more flexibility we have with our children's eating, the less often power struggles will develop. If parents are rigid about the evils of sugar or fat or carbs, their children may sneak these forbidden foods at a friend's house. This behavior can trigger more serious problems involving secrecy and shame about eating. Eating a wide range of foods—including bread, pasta, some fats, and desserts—imparts the message that food is not dangerous.

Allow children to regulate their own eating. Children are born self-regulating with their food. The less parents interfere in regulating their children's choices and quantity, the more children come to trust themselves—their inner hunger, their appetite, their satisfaction.

Enjoy family dinners. Create family dinners that are nutritious and plentiful, where people sit around and have conversations about thoughts and feelings. In the hustle and bustle of our everyday lives, it is sometimes hard to get together for family meals, yet they are so important. The family meal models a structure for children—meals have a beginning, middle, and end. Meals are a healthy antidote to the typical American method of grazing, snacking, and noshing all day long. Meals provide a variety of nutritious foods, unlike one-note, high-calorie, salty or sugary snack foods. And meals also give us an opportunity to just sit down! Sitting down to eat is fast becoming a rare behavior—eating on the run, standing over the sink, grazing in front of the open refrigerator, or wolfing down lunch in the car is common.

In contrast to our fast-food culture, the Spanish have a delightful expression, "estar de sobremesa," to describe the pleasure of taking the time after the meal is over to sit around the table chatting and enjoying one another's company.

Encourage emotions. The more we can encourage our children to express their emotions— hurt, anger, fear—the less they will need to turn to food to comfort themselves and relieve stress.

Accept your children. Parents must reconcile that children come in a variety of shapes and sizes, all of which are to be appreciated and celebrated. Some are naturally thin. Some are naturally heavier. Genetics plays a significant role in determining weight that no amount of restricting food will change. Let us love our children unconditionally as we ourselves long to be loved!

May our goal for ourselves and our children be: Sink your teeth into LIFE, not into excess food!

1   Research from the American Academy of Pediatrics demonstrates that boys are starting puberty six months to two years earlier than previously thought—the average is ten years for white and Hispanic boys, nine years for African-American boys. They are younger than ever, and are even *less* emotionally prepared for the changes of puberty. M. Herman-Giddens et al., "Secondary Sexual Characteristics in Boys: Data from the Pediatric Research in Office Settings Network," *Pediatrics*, 2012, 2011–3291. Previous research has identified a similar trend toward earlier puberty in girls, attributed by some experts to obesity and hormone-disrupting chemicals in the environment. F.M. Biro et al., "Pubertal Assessment Method and Baseline Characteristics in a Mixed Longitudinal Study of Girls," *Pediatrics*, 2010, 583–590.

2   In contrast, I remember with gratitude the night of my own prom. My father was working late, and I regretted not being able to show off for him how I looked in my fancy pink prom dress. When I returned from the prom late that night, I found a note from him, "Mama told me you looked beautiful tonight. I'm sorry I missed seeing you. Love, Papa." His note meant so much to me. I have kept it all these years later.

3   Victoria Secunda, *Women and Their Fathers: The Sexual and Romantic Impact of the First Man in Your Life* (Random House, 1993), 103.

4   A young girl comes for a consultation wearing very high stiletto heels, more appropriate for a disco than a therapist's office. "Wow," I comment, "those are really high heels!" She laughs and answers, "They're my 'knock me down and fuck me shoes.'" She is 15 years old.

Judith Warner, "Hot Tots, and Moms Hot to Trot," *New York Times*, March 17, 2007; http://query.nytimes.com/gst/fullpage html?res=9803E5D81F31F934A25750C0A9619C8B63&sc=&spon.

Diane Levin, Ph.D. and Jean Kilbourne, Ed.D., *So Sexy So Soon: The New Sexualized Childhood and What Parents Can Do to Protect Their Kids* (Ballantine Books, 2008).

5   Peggy Orenstein, *Cinderella Ate My Daughter* (Harper, 2012), 141.

6   Daniel Becker, *This Mean Disease: Growing Up in the Shadow of My Mother's Anorexia Nervosa* (Gürze Books, 2005). The poignancy of his experience is captured

in the prologue: "Mom's ashes are surprisingly heavy. Is it possible they could weigh more than she did when she died? After almost 30 years of anorexia nervosa, the cumulative effects are contained in a white porcelain urn."

7   "Thinheritance" explores the notion of how eating habits and body image may be passed down from parent to child. Schott's Vocab, *New York Times*, November, 4, 2009; http://schott.blogs.nytimes.com/2009/11/04/thinheritance/.

Dara-Lynn Weiss, in *The Heavy: A Mother, A Daughter, A Diet—A Memoir* (Ballantine Books, 2012) describes the abusive treatment she visits on her seven-year-old daughter to force the girl to lose weight. Ms. Weiss herself struggled with body image issues, diet pills, laxatives, and emetics to promote vomiting. Although she claims her strict, humiliating handling of her daughter was for her own good, readers will shudder at the "heavy"-handed approach, including publicizing the ordeal of her child in *Vogue* magazine. This is a cautionary tale of how *not* to help your daughter with eating issues:

"For Bea, the achievement [16-pound weight loss] is bittersweet. When I ask her if she likes how she looks now, if she's proud of what she's accomplished, she says yes. . . .   Even so, the person she used to be still weighs on her. Tears of pain fill her eyes as she reflects on her yearlong journey. 'That's still me,' she says of her former self. I'm not a different person just because I lost sixteen pounds.' I protest that, indeed, she is different. At this moment, that fat girl is a thing of the past. A tear rolls down her beautiful cheek. 'Just because it's in the past,' she says, 'doesn't mean it didn't happen.' "

8   The term "father hunger" was coined by Judith Viorst in *Necessary Losses* to describe the yearning that both girls and boys, men and women, experience for an absent or depriving father. Judith Viorst, *Necessary Losses* (Simon & Schuster, 1976), 74.

9   Charles M. Blow, "Remembrances of My Father," *New York Times*, June 18, 2011.

10   Dan Kindlon and Michael Thompson, *Raising Cain: Protecting the Emotional Life of Boys* (Random House, 2000), xix, 94, 95.

11   Kindlon, *Raising Cain*, 159.

12   Kindlon, *Raising Cain*, 116, 119.

13   Ellyn Satter, *Child of Mine: Feeding with Love and Good Sense* (Bull Publishing, 2000).

7. Sexual Abuse and Substance Abuse

Sadly, no book about eating disorders is complete without a discussion of sexual abuse. In my practice, about 50 percent of the men and women who come for therapy for emotional eating have been molested.

"It was my father's best friend." "It was my father." "It was my brother." "It was my mother's boyfriend." "It was my mother."

"And so I starved myself." "And so I ate." "And so I got fat." "And so I started using laxatives."

Sexual Abuse: A Family Affair

Sexual or physical abuse by a parent or family member inhibits the emotional growth of a child. The sacred innocence of the child is shattered. Abuse becomes a primary trigger of an eating disorder in a child or teen.

What is the connection between sexual abuse and developing an eating disorder? The victim of sexual abuse becomes plagued with guilt, shame, fear, anxiety, self-punishment, and rage. He or she seeks the soothing comfort, protection, and anesthesia that food offers.

Sexual abuse violates the boundaries of the self so dramatically that inner sensations of hunger, fatigue, or sexuality become difficult to identify. People who have been sexually abused may turn to food to relieve a wide range of different tension states that have nothing to do with hunger, because the betrayal they experienced has made them confused and mistrustful about their inner perceptions.

Survivors of sexual abuse often try to de-sexualize themselves. They hope this will protect them from sexual advances by others or even to wipe out their own sexual feelings which feel too threatening to deal with. They may work to make themselves very fat or very thin in an attempt to render themselves unattractive. Survivors may not be fully aware of how they manipulate food or their bodies to make themselves feel safer. Much of this behavior occurs unconsciously, behind the scenes, until therapy helps increase the person's awareness.

Some large men and women survivors actually fear losing weight because it will make them feel smaller and childlike, ushering in earlier memories of feeling defenseless that are difficult to cope with from when they were a child.

Other survivors obsessively diet, starve, or purge to make their bodies "perfect." Having a perfect body is their attempt to feel more powerful, invulnerable, and in control, so as not to re-experience the powerlessness they felt as children.

The ongoing impact of abuse cannot be minimized. In a recent court case, an 18- year-old girl, victimized by a community religious leader since she was 12, testified: "It takes years and years to heal, possibly to never fully recover. Personally, I feel the outcome of abuse is far worse than murder. With murder, the person is dead and it is final, while the person who was abused keeps dying day in and day out."

In addition to falling prey to eating disorders, all victims of sexual abuse are vulnerable to depression, substance abuse, post-traumatic stress disorder, and a profound mistrust of intimacy.

Sexual Abuse and Secrecy
Sexual abuse and emotional eating both contain one element in common: secrecy. Many eating disorder patients feel guilty about the

sexual abuse in their childhoods, believing they could have prevented it but chose not to because of some defect in themselves. They repress their secret and push it underground, and then distract and anesthetize themselves by emotional eating.

In some cases, children do not tell about their abuse because they do not realize at the time that anything wrong was happening. Those who are dependent on the abuser cannot risk upsetting the status quo. Often, children keep the abuse secret out of fear they will not be believed or because they were threatened or bribed to keep silent. A number of women patients have discussed sibling sexual abuse that occurred with their brothers.

There are many harmful forms of sexual abuse beyond overt touching. Covert abuse—a seductive, stimulating attitude by an adult—also wreaks damage. One father repeatedly bragged to his daughter about the size of his testicles and how he needed special large underwear to accommodate them. Another patient reported how her father and brother would forcefully hold her down and tickle her all over until she was gasping for breath.

Many eating disordered girls I have worked with speak with dismay of their father's scrutiny of one particular part of their body: her hair, her belly, her backside, her breasts. His intrusiveness, even when no touching is involved, leaves the girl feeling encroached upon and self-conscious. Many women with eating disorders reveal how their fathers called them tramps or whores when they began dating. One woman described how, starting at the age of 14, her father constantly hounded her as to whether she was still a virgin.

"After my parents divorced, my mother would get drunk and dance around the house in her nightgown," Donald described shamefully. "She scared me, but the worst part was I also got turned on. I began eating compulsively. I couldn't get the food in me fast enough. I never knew any other boy this happened to. What kind of family do I come from? There must be something wrong with us."

"My father never actually touched me," said Ava, a bulimic girl, "except with his eyes."

Whether the abuse is overt or covert, it damages a child's security and trust in the family and other relationships.

Post-Traumatic Stress Disorder

People with eating problems often suffer from symptoms of post-traumatic stress disorder (PTSD) without realizing the origins lie in sexual abuse. Post-traumatic stress is an emotional disorder resulting in recurrent anxiety, depression, a sense of being chronically "dead" inside, insomnia or nightmares, or experiencing a painful and heightened vigilance to one's surroundings. Some victims of post-traumatic stress also become involved in self-destructive behavior by forming repetitive abusive relationships, as well as losing themselves to drugs, alcohol, promiscuity, or self-mutilation.

Of course, none of these symptoms is absolute confirmation of abuse, but they are strong indicators of past sexual trauma. This is especially true if a person identifies several of these symptoms, since PTSD is usually a constellation of more than one warning sign. Connecting these symptoms to an actual event of sexual abuse, when possible, can be a validating experience, because then symptoms of inner turmoil begin to make sense.

Healing from Sexual Abuse

> *Now that my ladder's gone,*
> *I must lie down where all the ladders start*
> *In the foul rag and bone shop of the heart.*
> —W.B. Yeats

Being sexually abused is a nightmare of loneliness and fear and devastation. How can you heal from it?

Everyone's healing journey is unique to them, and everyone's healing time frame is different. The healing process begins with a willingness to reach out beyond yourself. The first step is to recount your experience to someone you trust who can help you go through the brunt of your pain, fear, and rage as it emerges. Because the experience of sexual abuse is about being out of control, you need to be in a safe setting where your feelings can reemerge and let loose. Releasing pain and guilt is not an intellectual experience, but something that comes from deep within the heart. This can be a difficult step because exposing your emotions can leave you feeling vulnerable, as if in a reenactment of the original trauma. Finding a compassionate therapist and/or a survivor's group can support this process. The healing process emerges slowly over time. It cannot be forced.

Although the media now covers the prevalence of sexual abuse more than ever before, this does not relieve the shame that many people feel about their own particular situation. If you have been a victim of incest, facing the abuse means facing not only the shame that you come from the kind of family where abuse is perpetrated, but also the rage that no one in your family protected you. Men who have been sexually abused as children, either by a male relative or by their mother, have distinct shame issues related to emotions of passivity and weakness.

Sometimes eating disorder patients feel strong guilt for having enjoyed the sexual contact with their abuser. Binge eating, purging, or starving then becomes their ongoing self-induced punishment. When we scratch the surface of the lives of these children, though, we discover that sexual abuse may have been the only real affection or caring they received. A child who is lonely or starved for affection may get pleasure from the attention, even if it is abusive. But the truth is that children are *never* to blame—they are *always* the victims. The only thing a child is guilty of is the innocent wish to be loved.

Confronting your shame, releasing your pain, and experiencing rage and guilt are part of the process of reclaiming your inner self as well as your sexual self. The need to detour your feelings through destructive eating will subside and slowly diminish when you are able to truly let yourself grieve for the little child you once were, who was betrayed.

This is the deepest part of recovery. Being able to feel sorrow for yourself, to cry, to view yourself with compassion, to acknowledge the loss of your innocence, to recognize the impact the abuse has caused are all milestones on the journey. Reliving the experiences of pain can set the stage for moving forward, gradually shedding the past, and reclaiming the wholeness that is inherently your right.

Daria had worked deeply and wholeheartedly on resolving her incest issues. The complication for her was that her abusive father was also her more loving parent. Daria's mother was cruel and unloving, while her father could often be appropriately affectionate and supportive. Daria had to contain and "digest" the contradiction that her father was both an abuser and, at times, a loving parent. It is so much easier when experiences are black and white but, like life itself, they often are not!

Painful residue remains for Daria, at times threatening to cloud her well-being. However, she created a tiny ritual to bring herself back into loving alignment whenever memories, anger, or bitterness threatened to surge up. "This is very powerful for me," explained Daria. "I take my hand and lift it up to my lips. I kiss my own hand with great love and tenderness and softness. Through this small gesture, I then feel restored by my own self-love!"

Daria also practiced a series of affirmations that included:

- Recovery is absolutely possible and achievable for me.
- I release and forgive myself for any responsibility I have accepted in the past for my abuse.
- My Dad (or the abuser(s) from the past) chose to hurt me. I will

not continue that legacy by hurting my own self in any way (food, relationships, drinking) but instead will practice self care.

• Offering myself daily compassion is necessary for my healing and growth.

• I commit to connecting to the child inside me today so we can play, laugh, and experience joy together.

• Feeling is healing; as I heal, I develop the ability to experience a wider range of emotions to enhance my health and connections to others.[1]

Group Therapy

Group treatment for women with abuse histories and eating disorders can be a powerful tool of recovery. Psychoanalyst Gwenn Nusbaum describes how in the context of an empathic therapy group, women help each other learn to negotiate the intense feelings of shame, guilt, desire, and hunger. In group, members learn to deal with "the delicate balance between too much and too little" as well as "not too hot, not too cold, not too distant, not too far" as they learn to respond to their own needs and to establish boundaries with others.[2]

Is Forgiveness Necessary to Heal?

Many abuse victims, as well as mental-health workers, believe that arriving at the point where you can forgive your abuser is the ultimate goal of recovery. Without achieving forgiveness, they claim, you are neither healed nor healthy.

Books on forgiveness exhort us to *Forgive and Forget; Unconditional Forgiveness: A Simple and Proven Method to Forgive Everyone; Let It Go: Forgive So You Can Be Forgiven; I Forgive You: Why You Should Always Forgive; Do Yourself a Favor . . . Forgive;* and *The Power of Forgiveness: How to Quickly Get Over the Past.* Counselors recommend a forgiveness formula and instruct us that "forgiveness is a choice, forgiveness is a gift, and you should strive for total forgiveness." The most damaging message of all is: "Unforgiveness is a learned behavior that can become a cancer of the soul that metastasizes if gone unchecked."

I refute this authoritarian notion about forgiveness. Forgiveness may indeed be part of recovery but *not* forgiving can also be a valid position. No one can tell you there is one right way to handle an abuse experience. Everyone needs to create a personal road map of recovery.

The outright assertion that, "You are not recovered unless you forgive your abuser" can actually be viewed as another form of abuse—psychological bullying and coercion, pressuring you as to how you should think and feel. Just as the abuser pressured and forced you to do his bidding.

Forgiveness is defined as a change of heart toward someone who has wronged you in which you overcome feelings of resentment and anger. But, in truth, forgiveness is not such a black or white concept. It may include a range of alternatives—from a genuine feeling of pardon to the victimizer on one hand to absolutely never forgiving on the other, with a continuum in between. And it may change over time.

In *The Courage to Heal*, the authors state, "Developing forgiveness for your abuser, or for the members of your family who did not protect you, is *not* a required part of the healing process. It is insulting to suggest to any survivor that she should forgive the person who abused her. This advice minimizes and denies the validity of her feelings. Yet the issue of forgiveness is one that will be pressed on you again and again by people who are uncomfortable with your rage. . . . You should never let anyone talk you into trading in your anger for the 'higher good' of forgiveness."[3]

I also think there is an important distinction between understanding and forgiving. You may understand the dynamics of the abuser and why he or she resorted to abuse. You may learn that the abuser also was a childhood victim. This is not the same as forgiveness, because understanding someone's behavior does not exonerate them. The slogan instructs, "To understand all is to forgive all." In my mind, a more accurate version would be, "To understand all is merely to understand all."

Chris Anderson, the executive director of MaleSurvivor.org, states, "I believe it is absolutely possible to be on the healing path without addressing whether or not we forgive those who have hurt us. If there is anyone that survivors need to be able to forgive it is *ourselves*. Many of us attack and blame ourselves for the dysfunction and destruction others brought into our lives. If we can let go of that pain, we are better able to live better and more satisfying lives. For those burdened by the pain of the past, it is a great challenge to live in the present. But it is by living in the present that we increase our chances of recovering. By living in the present we can better connect to people who give us more of what we need—hope and support—so that we can heal."[4]

If survivors on their own, without outside pressure, can *organically* arrive at a place in their hearts of being able to say, "I forgive you," it may well serve as a step toward healing. But forgiveness should not be demanded as the main component of recovery.[5]

Self-forgiveness, however, is a crucial component of recovery. Victims often worry they were complicit in allowing themselves to be abused; they do not fully appreciate their vulnerability and helplessness. After all, it is psychologically more protective to believe "I am a bad child" than to believe, for example, "my father is a bad father." Children need that father to protect them and cannot run the risk of losing him. They turn the "badness" on themselves. Therapy can help generate self-compassion for the untenable situation the victim found him/herself in.

Recovering from abuse includes any path that will lead you to feel whole and healthy, with compassion for yourself and the ability to be genuinely intimate with the people you love.

Eating Disorders and Substance Abuse

Why spend money on what is not bread,
and your labor on what does not satisfy?
Listen, listen to me, and eat what is good
and your soul will delight in the richest of fare.
                                        —Isaiah 55:2

Nothing is so bad that a few drinks won't make it worse.
                                        —AA slogan

Over the years, I have treated many people with both eating disorders and alcohol and drug addiction. My experience is borne out by statistics which show between 25 to 50 percent of anorexics, bulimics, and compulsive eaters abuse alcohol or drugs as well.[6]

The connection between eating disorders and substance abuse is complex:

- Some people abuse food, drugs, and alcohol simultaneously.
- Some people find their eating behavior worsens after they achieve sobriety from chemical dependency.
- For others, drinking and drugging worsens after progress is made in healing their eating disorder.
- Some people *intentionally* substitute drugs for food to help curtail their eating. Cocaine may be used because of its appetite-killing properties. Alcoholics, on the other hand, often turn to sweets and carbohydrates to curtail their drinking.

People will continue to substitute one addiction for another if the core issues that trigger their substance use are not addressed. Substituting addictions is like switching deck chairs on the Titanic.

No matter which chair you choose—you're still going down!

In the article, "Insatiable Hungers: Eating Disorders and Substance Abuse," Adrienne Ressler points out, "the word *satiate* comes from the Latin root *satis*, which means 'enough' and implies the capability of being fully satisfied. But for the thousands of individuals who experience the ravages of eating disorders and/or chemical dependency, their hungers are rarely satiated. For them, the high is never high enough, the number on the scale is never low enough, and the image in the mirror is never good enough. There is always a longing for more, better, faster—even instant gratification takes too long."[7]

People turn to substances or certain repetitive behaviors in an attempt to find peace of mind and soul, to find happiness and inner wholeness. But as Craig Nakken points out in his book, *The Addictive Personality*, "addiction is a process of buying into false and empty promises: the false promise of relief, the false promise of emotional security, the false sense of fulfillment, and the false sense of intimacy with the world. . . . The addict seeks serenity through a person, place, or thing."[8]

And, of course, this "serenity" is short-lived, the pain returns, perhaps now coupled with guilt and shame, and the addictive person again searches for relief with their particular substance. The cycle keeps going.

Once upon a time, addictions referred to alcoholism and drug abuse. Gone are those "good old days." Now we recognize people may struggle with a wide variety of addictions, including gambling, sex, the Internet, compulsive shopping, pornography, exercise, smoking, workaholic tendencies, shoplifting, self-mutilation, a series of abusive relationships, anger (rageaholics), and, of course, food. These addictions are all "hunger diseases," a person's attempt to regulate insatiable yearnings or unbearable agitation through consuming substances, people, or things.[9]

So if just about anything can be an addiction, what does that word really mean? I believe *any* substance or behavior can have the potential for compulsive craving. Some people are addicted to tattooing, body piercing, plastic surgery, or tanning ("tanorexia"). These practices are thought to stimulate the pleasurable release of endorphins in the brain which could explain, in part, their addictive potential.

Addiction refers to a person's:

- Physical dependence plus psychological obsession on a *substance* (smoking).
- Mental dependence on a repetitive *behavior* (gambling).
- Obsessive *thoughts* that a person feels powerless to control ("I'm fat and ugly and must lose weight).

Jacqueline gorged on five heads of lettuce with mustard every night.

Angela drank ten cups of coffee daily.

Lance chewed gum incessantly.

Tina developed an addiction to artificial sweeteners, "I started with five packs of Splenda in my coffee, then increased to ten. When that amount wasn't sufficient to satisfy my 'sweet tooth,' I needed to keep upping the ante. I could not satisfy that beast within me and started even sprinkling Splenda on all my foods—yogurt, fruit, vegetables. . . even tuna fish! That probably amounted easily to 60 to 80 fake sugar packs a day."

Iris, an anorexic middle-aged woman, began to compulsively drink the orange-flavored fiber supplement Citrucel. Frightened and feeling undeserving of nourishing herself with real food, she drank gallons of this liquid. "Why not just have orange juice, rather than artificially flavored methylcellulose?" I challenged her. Iris replied, "I still don't feel comfortable eating real food yet. I'm halfway on the road between not eating anything at all and allowing myself full nutrition. I consider Citrucel to be medicine so I can allow myself to have it."

I persisted, "But why are you filling up on a substance that is not even food? It sounds like you're trying to train yourself to survive in case there is no real food to be had." Iris's face turned gray, and she slowly responded, "My mother told me when she was in Bergen-Belsen, the concentration camp in Germany, they had nothing to drink at all. My grandmother coaxed her, 'Bend down. Drink the mud. At least it's something.' My mother described how she scooped up the mud and swallowed it. I realize now that's the same as me. My Citrucel is the mud I'm trying to live on. Maybe I'm trying to prove to myself that I too could have the strength to survive on nothing like they did. Or maybe I need to honor the suffering of my family by repeating what they had to go through."

Checking e-mail compulsively, exercising despite injury, and immersing oneself so deeply in work that family obligations or vacations become an unwanted intrusion can all be examples of addictive behavior. In characteristic bulimic behavior, Eva "binged" on $4,000 worth of clothes only to "purge" the next day by returning them to the store.

These addictions help people relieve stress, alter an uncomfortable mood, numb emotional turmoil, escape from reality, relieve depression or anxiety, isolate from people or responsibilities. Although Jacqueline's staying home and bingeing on lettuce and mustard every night is obviously not as destructive as using crack cocaine, it still interfered with her living life with real satisfaction. Rather than coming to terms with a painful divorce and her fears of creating a new social life for herself, Jacqueline retreated to her apartment, using the "substance" of lettuce. This compulsion diminished her living in the real world—even though it was just lettuce!

Why does someone develop both eating disorders and substance abuse?

The media propagates the notion that happiness, success, and self-worth are dependent on slenderness. Anorexia is glamorized. This undue pressure to be thin leads many women into substance abuse—licit or illicit. Papers presented at the Eighth International Conference on Eating Disorders in 1995 showed that a significant number of women abuse cocaine for the express purpose of losing weight, because appetite suppression is a major side effect of this drug. Many women also turn to cigarette smoking to alleviate hunger.

Vulnerability to anxiety or depression causes people to turn to food, alcohol, and/or drugs as an escape. Addictions and eating disorders are misguided attempts to fill up an inner psychic emptiness.

Current research indicates genetics or other complex biological processes may give rise to an eating disorder, drug, and/or alcohol abuse. Neurotransmitters, such as dopamine, are chemicals in the brain responsible for pleasure. A deficiency of these chemicals is linked to carbohydrate cravings, depression, anxiety, obsessive disorders, bulimia, and drug and alcohol abuse.

People with eating disorders and substance abuse often come from families with these same illnesses. This implies that either addiction is hereditary (nature) or families, by their example, model lifestyles to their children which include disordered eating or chemical abuse (nurture). Sometimes it is a combination of both nature and nurture.

If a person suffers sexual or physical abuse in childhood, the trauma of betrayal often leads to the abuse of mood-altering substances to quell the pain, fear, guilt, and self blame that can follow.

Drugs of Choice
Let's look at the substances—both legal and illegal—that eating disordered people might abuse in addition to food.

Caffeine
Caffeine is often abused by those with eating disorders to fill themselves up and camouflage their hunger. Caffeine is also a diuretic, and people with eating disorders confuse temporary fluid loss with actual weight loss. Many of my eating disorder patients rely on their coffee,

lattes, cappuccinos, mochaccinos, frappuccinos, and caffeinated soft drinks to suppress their appetite and get them through the day without eating. Energy drinks designed to quell hunger due to their high caffeine content—Rockstar Energy, Monster Energy, Red Bull, Full Throttle—continue to hit the market, despite their implication in heart attacks and even deaths.

Ultimately, caffeine does not help weight loss, is not nutritious, and can cause insomnia. Large amounts of caffeine give people the jitters, a troublesome side effect, especially for those with anxiety disorders![10]

Alcohol

Drinking has been described as "A love story. Yes: this is a love story. It's about passion, sensual pleasure, deep pulls, lust, fears, yearning hungers. It's about needs so strong they're crippling. [Recovery is] about saying goodbye to something you can't live without.

"I loved the way drink made me feel, and I loved its special power of deflection, its ability to shift my focus away from my own awareness of self and onto something else, something less painful than my own feelings."[11]

The recovering alcoholics in my practice tend to be compulsive overeaters and bulimics. Anorexics generally do not consume alcohol for fear of the fattening calories and because of their "commitment" to restriction. Scientific studies have demonstrated a genetic, biochemical connection between alcoholism, bulimia, and depression.

Because alcohol is a sedative, someone with an eating disorder may turn to drinking to take the edge off anxiety. "Liquid courage" may help a person feel more relaxed in social situations. But alcohol is not nutritious, is highly caloric, and, most of all, is a depressant. The very depression the person hoped the alcohol would relieve can backfire, and one's depression worsens.

Laxatives and diuretics

As we discussed in chapter 3, laxative and diuretic abuse is a type of bulimic behavior. Compulsive overeaters and bulimics are especially prone to misuse them, believing they will cause weight loss. The body appears to lose weight, but it is merely water loss which immediately returns after these substances are discontinued.

Laxative abuse can cause physical problems with the colon as well as emotional tension because of the need to manipulate one's schedule to run to the bathroom at a moment's notice. A subgroup of laxative abusers are people who consume large amounts of fiber in bran muffins and bran cereal and drink laxative teas in extreme amounts in the false hope they will evacuate excess calories.

Over-the-counter diet pills

Women's magazines often feature an array of ads claiming quick weight-loss through nonprescription pills. Drug stores and health food stores carry weight-loss pills in abundance. Some pills are touted as "natural," as if that means they are always safe. Natural does not necessarily mean safe; after all, poison ivy is natural too! The dangerous health consequences of diet pill abuse include high blood pressure, abnormal heart rhythms, tremors, thickening of the heart muscle, and kidney damage.

Prescription pills

Sleeping pills, anti-anxiety medication, and pain killers, although legal and available by a doctor's prescription, are frequently abused by eating disorder individuals. As we often see in the media, many people die from overdosing on *legal* prescription pills.[12]

Tobacco

The nicotine in tobacco is an appetite suppressant that can increase metabolism as much as 10 percent in females. It is not unusual for girls with eating disorders to start smoking in an effort to control their appetite. Of course, the health consequences of long-term cigarette smoking can be devastating.

Marijuana

Marijuana is often smoked for the high it produces, although people with eating disorders may shun it for fear of its stimulating effect on the appetite. The beguiling names of marijuana promise relief for vulnerable individuals from life's stress and strain: Purple Haze, Northern Lights, Laughing Grass, God Bud, Champagne.

Amphetamines and cocaine

Amphetamines, also known as speed, are the same drugs diet doctors prescribed decades ago for overweight patients. The pills were eventually found to cause physiological dependence, rapid heartbeat, and insomnia, and their use was discontinued. Crystal meth, an illegal and much more powerful form of amphetamine, suppresses appetite very strongly. People who use this extremely dangerous drug sometimes go days without eating. Some women, especially in rural and working-class populations, may use crystal meth as an appetite suppressant. Although I personally have not seen this addiction in my practice in the New York City area, therapists in other areas, especially the west, southeast, and and southwest, may see female patients who use meth. It is cheaper, more long-lasting, and even more addictive than cocaine. Meth can be snorted, smoked, injected, or inhaled. Similarly, those with eating disorders often resort to illegal cocaine, another psychomotor stimulant, because it suppresses appetite and gives the body a boost of energy. Cocaine is highly addictive and can cause psychosis, respiratory failure, and heart attacks.

Similarities between Eating Disorders and Substance Abuse

Both eating disorders and substance abuse have a mood-altering effect. Food, like alcohol and drugs, can be used to comfort, to soothe, to kill pain, to anesthetize, to sedate anxiety, to relieve tension, or to stimulate and enliven a depressed mood.

Denial is the hallmark of both disorders. People refuse to admit that their substance use and eating disorder has a detrimental physical or emotional effect on them.

Addictions, like eating disorders and substance abuse, are diseases of isolation—the person and progressively withdraws from relationships or work obligations. This is due to the increasing amount of time needed to *get* food or drugs, *consume* food or drugs, and *recover* from their effects. (The aftermath of gorging on large quantities of food or repeatedly purging is similar to a hangover from drinking. It leaves one in a depleted, bloated, dehydrated state). Even the emaciated anorexic isolates, the better to exercise frantically in secret or to claim she has previously eaten when she has not.

Loss of control and unsuccessful efforts to regain control are similar for the emotional eater and the substance abuser. Both groups make pacts with themselves, "I'll quit tomorrow" or "I'll begin my diet on Monday." They vow to double-up on their willpower. The truth is, many addicted people *can* abstain for periods of time, but only temporarily. The key issue for the addicted person is they cannot *stay stopped*. Willpower can help a person halt destructive behavior temporarily, but it does not prevent relapse. Until people make the *internal* changes to sustain recovery, they will continue to relapse. Recovery is an *inside* job. Mark Twain, describing his own battle with tobacco, once quipped, "Quitting smoking is easy—I've done it hundreds of times!"

Both chemically dependent and eating disorder people often feel shame and guilt at the very core of their being. This becomes intensified as they see themselves resorting to any means to get their fix—lying, inventing alibis, covering up, stealing food or money.

Andrea, a binge eater from an alcoholic family, confessed how she would sneak cookies into the bathroom to hide her eating from her boyfriend, John. I encouraged her to come out of the "john" and eat in front of John to break the ongoing cycle of eating, shame, and secrecy that she perpetuated by hiding.

The compulsion to hide and sneak is so strong with addicts that Ilene described hiding food in her bathroom hamper—even though she lived alone!

Chemically dependent people develop an increased tolerance for their drug. As their body becomes habituated to the drug, they then require larger amounts to achieve the same effect.

It is debatable whether eating disorder patients develop an increased tolerance for food, but I do believe the action of bingeing, purging, or starving often takes on a life of its own, spiraling out of control in an increasingly progressive cycle.

Impaired intimacy is another similarity. Both the chemically dependent person and the emotional eater believe that trusting their substance is safer than trusting people. No human relationship complies with one's needs for instant gratification so absolutely.

Both eating disorder patients and substance abusers suffer an increased incidence of depression or anxiety disorders. Ironically, food, alcohol, and drugs then become self-medication, which perpetuates the vicious cycle."

Differences between Substance/Alcohol Abuse and Eating Disorders

We must have food to live, while drugs or alcohol are not required to sustain life.

Food is always legal. Although we can debate whether double-fudge-chocolate-decadent-black-out cake should be outlawed, the truth is food is always legal. Of course, many drugs and substances are also legal—alcohol, prescription pills, over-the-counter diet pills, laxatives, diuretics, tobacco. However, many of our most addictive and toxic substances are illegal— amphetamines, co-caine, marijuana, heroin.

Food is an important part of most celebrations of life. Food is the cheapest, most socially sanctioned, most available mood-altering drug on the market.

Although overeating may be more socially acceptable than drug or alcohol abuse, a tremendous stigma is attached to being a fat, compulsive eater. Society, more often than not, frowns on compulsive overeating, viewing it as evidence of moral weakness and lack of willpower. Rarely is it acknowledged that overweight or obesity may be the result of genetics.

Anorexia is the only eating disorder that engenders sympathy. The anorexic is viewed as a troubled victim with a terrible, life-threatening affliction. Unlike any other addiction, anorexia may also stimulate envy in others. Many eating disorder sufferers wish to become anorexic and feel disappointed when they are unable to starve themselves to that coveted size 0.

People with eating disorders have more body image disturbances. Underlying all eating disorders is significant anxiety about being fat. Alcoholics or drug-addicted people do not experience this fear of fat.

Various substances disrupt brain functioning and affect eating behavior in different ways. Nicotine stimulates metabolism. Alcohol, amphetamines, cocaine, and caffeine reduce hunger, and so are used as an appetite suppressant. Marijuana, on the other hand, promotes food cravings. Heroin and opiates interfere with nutritional absorption and can be lethal.

Food is always ingested by mouth, while drugs can be swallowed (pills, alcohol), snorted (cocaine, meth), smoked (marijuana, meth), injected (heroin, meth), inhaled (glue, tobacco, meth). The only exception to this rule is the laxative abuser who recruits the other end of the digestive system to evacuate food.

The seductive names of many substances enhance their allure. One patient described her "love affair" with the laxative Correctol. She fantasized that by forcibly evacuating her food, she could "correct all" of her life's many troubling problems. One alcoholic patient binged on Southern Comfort; a binge eater gorged on brownies named Magic Mommy, while another indulged in the brand of cookies called Almost Home. And I, as a little girl, feasted on Good & Plenty candy. The name was so very reassuring to me, even though I disliked licorice!

Abstinence from drugs and alcohol is clearly defined—to completely halt their use. Since food is obviously necessary to live, abstinence for the eating disorder person is open to varying interpretations. Some recovery groups define abstinence as following a predetermined, structured food plan or the elimination of sugar and flour from one's diet. Others define recovery as learning to eat when hungry and stop when full.

Rather than trying to define abstinence, I believe true recovery from an eating disorder involves:

1. Eliminating the behaviors of starving, bingeing, purging, chronic dieting, and body hatred.
2. An increased capacity to tolerate and cope with stress.
3. The management/resolution of obsessive thoughts about weight and food.
4. Developing a more harmonious, enjoyable relationship with food and exercise.
5. Enhanced intimacy and nourishment from people.

Treating Eating Disorders and Substance Abuse

All eating disorders contain multiple causes, multiple physical and emotional effects, and multiple solutions. When drugs and alcohol are added to the mix with an eating disorder, the treatment plan for recovery becomes more complex. Sometimes in treating one addiction, another addiction may flare up.

Amanda described her predicament, "The minute I got out of alcohol rehab and got sober, my overeating got worse. I was a binge eater since I was a young teenager. I thought I had conquered that compulsion. But then it came back to haunt me in sobriety."

Fighting two addictions at the same time is not uncommon. Diana came to therapy because of a 14-year nightly pattern of drinking a bottle or more of wine and gorging on cookies and ice cream. During the day, Diana functioned adequately as an insurance claims investigator. But her evenings were filled with loneliness and deep anxiety.

During the course of our work together, we created a four-point treatment plan for Diana to tackle both her eating/drinking abuse: (1) We established a regular and structured eating pattern of three meals daily with three to four snacks. The pattern was designed to give her something organized and concrete to hold onto when the loneliness of her evening felt chaotic and overwhelming. (2) Diana joined a women's eating support group and discussed her bingeing and drinking for the first time with others. (3) We explored the severe emotional and sexual abuse she had experienced as a little girl, which made her deeply mistrustful of people. She began taking antidepressant medication to reduce her agitation so she could better handle her daily responsibilities.

Over a period of time, these interventions led to a complete resolution of her nighttime drinking and a marked decrease in her bingeing, anxiety, and depression. By the age of 40, Diana had developed far more self-confidence, found a trustworthy partner, and adopted a baby girl.

Alcohol and bingeing were Diana's way to self-medicate her loneliness. The nourishment she received in therapy, the support from the women in the group, and the prescribed medication all provided a secure safety net for Diana. In time, she made great progress in working through her deep-seated issues of deprivation and betrayal which were the root cause of her food and alcohol abuse.

Therapists must always explore a range of healing strategies custom-tailored to each person with a double addiction. *Each person's problem is as unique as a fingerprint and requires an individualized intervention for his or her specific struggles. One size does not fit all.*

Allan also had a double addiction, but with a different set of issues than Diana. A 33-year-old gay man, Allan came to therapy for treatment of his depression. He also admitted to bulimia, but was reluctant to work on this. Mostly, he spoke about his disappointment with his boyfriend, as well as neglect during his childhood. Allan's parents divorced when he was two, moved to different states, and shuttled Allan between them until his father was sent to jail for a white-collar crime. As he purged his sadness and grief and thrashed out these experiences in treatment, Allan experienced temporary relief from his bulimia. But invariably he could not sustain the work we had done and would have a bulimic relapse. I was not sure why.

Then, in one session, Allan described a frightening experience from the previous weekend. Coming home from a party at 2 a.m., he had fallen asleep on a New York City subway train, missed his stop, and woke up in the middle of the night at the end of the line in a dangerous neighborhood.

This incident told me indirectly what Allan had kept secret. I suspected he had been drinking heavily and then passed out. Allan had previously denied alcohol use, although both his parents were alcoholics (as well as both stepparents). When I confronted him about his drinking, he admitted he hid it from me out of fear he would have to give it up. Recognizing his drinking had put him in a potentially dangerous situation helped break through his denial. He finally agreed to enter a rehab facility, committed to Alcoholics Anonymous meetings, and increased his therapy to twice a week. His bulimia subsided. He began pursuing a professional career for the first time in his life and eventually married a man he met in AA. The ongoing community of support of AA and his continued in-depth psychotherapy has provided Allan with a secure environment and a second-chance family.

Codependent Relationships

It is not unusual for an eating disordered woman to become involved with a partner with addictions. This is often a repetition of her family dynamics where early relationships were fraught with addiction. Also, being involved with someone with substance abuse helps her hide her own food abuse as she focuses on her mate's problems.

Sometimes the codependent person craves the chaos and dramatic crises in her life because they release a surge of adrenaline and endorphins. It is as if she becomes addicted to the rushes of her own body chemicals. As Whitney Houston said before she died of a lethal combination of alcohol and prescription pills, "My *husband* was my ongoing drug."

Vanessa used drugs recreationally as a teenager, as did her brother, Vincent, who became addicted. When Vanessa was 15, Vincent died of an overdose. Years later, Vanessa came to treatment for her binge eating disorder and obesity. Although she no longer used drugs after her brother's death, her life continued to be intertwined with addicts, as is the case for many eating disordered people.

Vanessa had married Ian, an alcoholic and drug addict in recovery. She steadfastly maintained her eating disorder throughout the marriage, until her husband relapsed and died of a drug overdose. Vanessa then finally recognized how her binge eating, obesity, and prediabetes were slowly eroding her health. Fearful she would not be healthy enough to take care of her children alone now that Ian was dead, Vanessa broke through her denial and sought therapy. Vanessa also began attending Overeaters Anonymous meetings.

Four months after Ian's death, Vanessa fell in love with her husband's best friend. She had known him for many years—he also was a recovering drug addict. Shortly into their relationship, Vanessa found Raymond in his apartment, foaming at the mouth and near death from a drug overdose. She called an ambulance in time to save his life. When I asked her quite pointedly how she had arranged to involve herself with *two* active addicts, she shamefully admitted that she felt superior to them. "After all," Vanessa said, "I only have an eating disorder. I may be fat, but at least drug addicts seem to like me!"

Exploring her sense of inadequacy enabled Vanessa to examine her history with codependent relationships and face her long-buried grief about her brother's death and her anger at her parents for ignoring all the warning signs. In a poignant session, Vanessa described how at the age of 12, she looked up "therapists" in the phone book with the hope of getting help for Vincent.

In time, she was able to directly face her pain and grief, rather than abusing food to shore up her shaky sense of self. Vanessa joined one of the women's eating support groups I lead and found ongoing support with Overeaters Anonymous. Raymond has entered a rigorous methadone program that offers them family therapy.

Diana, Allan, and Vanessa used food and substances to distract, detour, deny, and divert their emotional problems. They overcame their addictions because they took that first difficult but essential step toward recovery: *They admitted they were powerless over their food and substance abuse, and their lives had become unmanageable.* Recognizing the unmanageability of their lives prompted them to seek the help they needed and deserved.

The Treatment Plan

Cross addictions can have significant health risks, including death. It was a lethal combination of cocaine, Xanax, Valium, and alcohol that led to Whitney Houston's death at age 48 in 2012. Recently, a young woman, Jessica, came for a consultation. She was taking Ecstasy and hoodia (an ineffective herbal appetite suppressant) and was suffering from bulimia, alcohol abuse, and depression. I hospitalized her so that she could be detoxed and medically stabilized before any further treatment program was begun.

A multidisciplinary treatment that integrates help for both the addiction and disordered eating holds the greatest promise for solid recovery. Six types of treatment approaches for eating disorders plus substance abuse have been shown to be effective, alone or in combination.

1. Hospitalization. A patient who has anorexia or bulimia may be at significant risk for dehydration, starvation, and electrolyte imbalance which can lead to serious health complications and sometimes death. Similarly, substance abusers may need hospitalization to detoxify from their drug. Once a patient is medically stabilized, further treatment can begin.

2. 12-step recovery groups. Perhaps the most solid foundations for the recovery of substance abusers who are also eating disordered are the 12-step programs of Alcoholics Anonymous, Narcotics Anonymous, and Overeaters Anonymous. The ongoing emotional and spiritual journey that these fellowships provide bolsters the healing of addicted people and provides strategies of how to cope with stress without the crutch of substances. Bill B., author of *Compulsive Overeater*, describes addiction: "the problem is emotional, the symptom is physical, the solution is spiritual."[13]

The belief in a "higher power"—be it God, nature, one's best inner wisdom, Good Orderly Direction (G.O.D.), the still quiet voice within, the soul, the self—can provide deep inner comfort to the recovering person. No longer do recovering people have to fight and struggle with their own will. They can learn to surrender to a healing spiritual power greater than themselves.

3. *Cognitive-behavioral therapy (CBT).* This approach attempts to correct unhealthy habits and the distorted thinking patterns that keep a person stuck. Becoming aware of negative thoughts and behaviors that trigger disordered behavior is a key step toward substituting supportive alternatives. This awareness increases our consciousness to pause, reflect, and make different choices.

4. *Pharmacological intervention.* Addictions, depression, eating disorders, anxiety, obsessive-compulsive behaviors, social phobia, bipolar disorder, ADHD, panic attacks all have a biochemical as well as an emotional basis. Medications prescribed by a psychiatrist or physician can help alleviate these symptoms. This, in turn, supports the client's ability to deepen the commitment to working through psychological issues.

5. *Psychotherapy.* Psychotherapy is a most powerful channel for healing. Crucial to any successful therapy—no matter what the approach—is the healing relationship with the therapist. In order to change and grow, the recovering person needs to feel listened to, accepted for his or her genuine self, guided, supported, challenged and respectfully regarded. When a person can attach to a caring, loving person—such as a therapist or the people in a recovery group—the need to attach to food and substances will ebb as he learns to develop a supportive relationship with his very own self.

Some therapists insist their patients stop using/abusing as a prerequisite to begin therapy. Unless there is an immediate health risk, I find it more helpful to work in collaboration with the patient toward understanding the meaning of her relationship with the drug and how she hoped it would help her. This engages the person in a working alliance with the therapist rather than becoming adversaries. If the therapist demands abstinence at the outset of treatment, patients may want to comply but wind up rebelling by secretly using their substances or abruptly dropping out of treatment before they get the help they need.

6. *Combination therapies.* A blended approach of cognitive, psychological, behavioral, nutritional, and pharmacological methods provides the strongest support for ongoing, sustained recovery.

As we see, there are many paths to recovery. There is no "one-right-way." Father Leo Booth, addictions expert, writes, "Roads to recovery are as distinct and unique as the individuals who travel them. Some people grab onto recovery and never let go. Others struggle with relapse, multiple addictions, or chronic depression. Many people find it easier to stop all of their addictions at once. Others take it one compulsion at a time; alcoholics may get sober, then tackle their eating disorder, then smoking or codependency. . . . Look at the immense variety in our stories, how creative we were in practicing our dysfunctions. That same diversity and creativity go into recovery."[14]

Our goal for the eating disordered and chemically dependent person: To help you contact your inner vigor and vitality and sink your teeth into LIFE, not into mood-altering substances!

1   Adapted from Howard Fradkin, Ph.D., Co-Chairperson, MaleSurvivor Weekends of Recovery; www.MaleSurvivor.Org.

2   Gwen Nusbaum, "Interest or Intrusion? Navigating the Thin Line and What is in Between in a Psychoanalytic Group for Women with Incest Traumas and Eating Disorders," *GROUP*, vol. 30, no. 4, December 2006.

3   Ellen Bass and Laura Davis, *The Courage to Heal* (HarperCollins, 1994), 160–162.

4   Chris Anderson, "Forgiveness," MaleSurvivor.Org, October 3, 2012.

5   A colleague of mine, Ellen S. Daniels, LCSW, suggests this interpretation of forgiveness:
    Patients often ask their therapists, "Do I have to forgive him/her/them in order to move on?" I've come to the conclusion that perhaps one answer is succinctly contained in the following quote from the movie, *Grosse Pointe Blank:* "Some say forgive and forget. I say forget about forgiving and just accept. And get the hell out of town." When I tell this quote to patients, we look at "getting the hell out of town"

as a metaphor for remembering, feeling, and working through. And then moving on with life, aiming to find the basic sense of stable well-being that is, after all, the goal of all good therapy. So, yes, people can recover without forgiveness. Understanding/accepting may be exactly enough.

6   Joseph A. Califano, "Food for Thought: Substance Abuse and Eating Disorders," a report from the National Center on Addiction and Substance Abuse (CASA) at Columbia University, 2004. This study was the first comprehensive examination of the link between substance abuse and eating disorders. It reveals that up to one-half of individuals with eating disorders abuse alcohol or illicit drugs, compared to 9 percent of the general population. Conversely, up to 35 percent of alcohol or illicit drug abusers have eating disorders, compared to 3 percent of the general population.

7   Adrienne Ressler, MA, LMSW, CEDS, "Insatiable Hungers: Eating Disorders and Substance Abuse," *Social Work Today,* July/August 2008, vol. 8, 30.

8   Craig Nakken, *The Addictive Personality: Understanding the Addictive Process and Compulsive Behavior* (Hazelden, 1996).

9   Raymond Battegay, *The Hunger Diseases* (Jason Aronson, 1991).

10   The *New York Times* reports more than 13,000 emergency room visits were associated with energy drinks in 2009, and the drinks have been implicated in heart attacks, convulsions, and death. Barry Meier, "More Emergency Visits Linked to Energy Drinks," *New York Times,* January 11, 2013; http://www.nytimes.com/2013/01/12/business/more-emergency-room-visits-linked-to-energy-drinks-report-says.html and Barry Meier, "F.D.A. Posts Injury Data for 3 Drinks," *New York Times,* November 15, 2012; http://www.nytimes.com/2012/11/16/business/scrutiny-of-energy-drinks-grows.html?_r=0.

11   Caroline Knapp, *Drinking: A Love Story* (Bantam Dell, 2005).

12   Overdoses of prescription pain medications are up 90 percent since 1999 and accidental ODs now kill more Americans than car crashes. Every year, nearly 15,000 people die from overdoses involving prescription pain killers—more than those who die from heroin and cocaine combined. Centers for Disease Control, National Center for Injury Prevention and Control, Division of Unintentional Injury Prevention, "Prescription Painkiller Overdoses in the U.S.," February 15, 2012; http://www.cdc.gov/Features/VitalSigns/PainkillerOverdoses/index.html.
     "More than 15,000 Americans now die annually after overdosing on prescription painkillers. Drug overdoses are now the single largest cause of accidental death in America. . .   . The legality of prescription painkillers makes their abuse harder

to tackle." "Prescription for Addiction: America's Deadliest Drug Epidemic," *Wall Street Journal*, October 6, 2012.

13   Bill B., *Compulsive Overeater: The Basic Text for Compulsive Overeaters* (Hazelden, 1988).

14   Father Leo Booth, MTh, CAC, CEDS, "Many Paths to Recovery," *Journal of the International Association of Eating Disorders Professionals*, Summer 1999.

8. From Gridlock to Growth: Confronting Obstacles to Change

> If we wait for the moment when everything, absolutely everything, is ready, we shall never begin.
>
> —Ivan Turgenev

"I'm willing to do *anything* to lose weight," announces Julie, a new client.

She pauses. I wait expectantly.

"Except eat right and exercise," she adds.

We laugh heartily at the shared recognition that the effort to eat right and exercise is so much easier said than done.

Motivation and Willingness

Julie's candid admission touches on an intriguing aspect of resolving an eating disorder—the role of motivation. What is motivation? How do you get it? How do you sustain it?

The dictionary defines motivation as "some inner drive, impulse, intention that causes a person to act in a certain way; an incentive; a goal." I would add that motivation is the fuel that impels people to change.

Even the Bible refers to motivation problems: "I do not understand my own actions. For I do not do what I want, but I do the very thing I hate"(Romans 7:15). This description reveals the very core of motivation problems—we are divided against our self. The head wants one thing, the appetites want something else. Julie wants to lose weight but another part of her doesn't want to make the effort. It's as if she is in a civil war with her very own self.

People are always conflicted about change, even change for the better. Change is disconcerting and disorienting and unknown. Many people try to ignore and jump over their resistance to change by attempting to commit to a grand dramatic project, "I will not eat any desserts anymore." "I will only eat 1,000 calories." "I will not eat bread or pasta ever again." These rigid proclamations are bound to fail because they are not sustainable. Rigidity always backfires. Rather than recommending anything unsustainable, I asked Julie what *small* step she might like to try toward improving her eating patterns. Julie suggested adding a salad to her daily lunch. This was a great suggestion, because rather than depriving herself by taking food away, Julie chose to *add* something enriching to her meal. That the idea came from her made it all the better. Julie could not solve her whole eating problem at once, but she did have the willingness to make one small change. If we can reduce a problem to its "bite-size" components, recovery is much less daunting.

Julie's salad may seem like an insignificant step. But the truth is that healing is a process composed of small links on a chain, one leading to another. *No change is too small.* This is especially so because if a person can successfully accomplish even a small change, this can lead to more hopeful feelings which, in turn, will generate further progress. Making a commitment to short-term change can build momentum for long-term progress.

Suzanne had been bulimic most of her adult life. She described a typical day: after work, she would drive to a grocery store, buy a cake, and gorge on it while driving home. Once home, she would make herself throw up. Then feeling utterly disgusted with herself, she would drive out again, buy some more cake, and throw up again.

"I must totally change my behavior right now," Suzanne declared with ferocity and self-hate. Given that she had been bulimic for so many years, I doubted that she could curtail her bingeing and purging overnight.

I suggested an alternative: She should buy her cake as usual, drive to a quiet block and park, and then calmly savor the cake, rather than wolfing it down while driving. I added, "Before tearing into the cake, give it a kiss and thank it for helping you cope with whatever anxiety you are feeling at that time. Then relish it slowly and let it stay inside your tummy."

Suzanne said, "That sounds weird." But the following week she reported several peaceful rendezvous with the cake. Self-loathing and yelling at herself had not helped motivate her to stop gorging and purging. A shift in attitude did. My suggestion enabled her to realize that devouring the cake was her way of comforting and taking care of herself. It did not mean she was a bad person. She developed more self-compassion and self-acceptance—and with that came hope. Slowly and gently, she became more motivated to make increasingly supportive changes.

Strategies to encourage your own motivation include:
- Recognize it is normal to feel ambivalence about making any change in your life. After all, the status quo is familiar and predictable.
- Identify the trigger that provokes you to overeat, purge, or starve: Comfort? Companionship? Release of anger?
- Acknowledge the price you pay for on-going hurtful eating behavior, both in terms of physical consequences and lowered self-esteem.
- If you decided to change, what do you think would work for you? What would be your first step? Respectfully consult with yourself.

- What will you do to support yourself with the process of change if things get tough? Think about what may have worked for you in the past.
- You don't have to tackle your whole eating problem at once. No dramatic upheavals required. Begin with, "I Will Do Just One Thing Differently." Drink more water during the day. Or exercise an extra five minutes. Or, like Julie, eat a daily salad. These caring alterations in your behavior will communicate to your brain you are ready to begin to change. Keep it simple. One step at a time.

Change is a process of stops and starts. As one of my clients said, "It doesn't matter how many times I've fallen off the wagon. What matters is how many times I get back up!" What will drive your motivation forward is an abiding compassion for yourself.

Identifying Personal Roadblocks

Faith is taking the first step, even when you don't see the whole staircase.

—Dr. Martin Luther King, Jr.

Let's explore the most frequent roadblocks to growth in order to prepare and support your healing work. The garden needs to be weeded and raked before the seeds are planted and watered.

Obstacles to change include:

- Denial about your eating problems.
- Ambivalence and conflict about whether you really want to change.
- Fear of success.

Denial

"My parents forced me to come for therapy, but I don't want to be here. There's nothing wrong with me," stated Miriam, a 16-year-old girl weighing 76 pounds.

"My wife insisted I come here, but I don't want to be here. There's nothing wrong with me," stated Kevin, a 43–year-old man with diabetes and weighing 325 pounds.

"My girlfriend made me come here because she hears me throwing up after dinner a lot of nights, but I don't want to be here. There's nothing wrong with me," stated Patricia, a 32-year-old woman with a two-year problem of bulimia.

Denial is the common denominator of all addictions. It is a formidable obstacle that can prevent us from resolving emotional eating. Denial is a tricky defense mechanism because it tells us everything is fine, despite strong evidence to the contrary. When someone is bulimic, anorexic, a binge eater, or an alcoholic, gambler, cigarette smoker, or drug addict, he or she may often not be able to admit the seriousness of the disorder. To admit that your behavior is self-destructive is the very first step that leads to recovery. To continue to deny is to continue to stay stuck.

A favorite cartoon of mine illustrates how we may justify and deny our own hurtful behavior:

A husband comes into the kitchen to find his wife bingeing on a gallon of ice cream and says, "Why are you eating all that ice cream? What about the diet you keep saying you're going to start?"

She responds: "I read how scientists say that eventually the sun will fry the earth, so what's the point of dieting?"

The husband points out, "I think that's not going to happen for a few billion years."

And the wife answers morosely, "Oh well, I a ready opened the ice cream" and keeps on bingeing.

Denial is not always a harmful defense mechanism. If we go to the dentist for a root canal or to the doctor for a medical procedure, it is helpful to protect ourselves by saying, "This is probably no big deal. It will be over soon enough." It is healthy to want to guard ourselves from pain. But when our behavior becomes self-destructive, it is time to admit the truth.

People turn to bingeing, purging, or starving because they fear the pain of confronting their feelings directly. What reinforces denial is that emotional eating may be one of the strongest sources of pleasure and satisfaction in a person's life. And common to all people in denial is their reluctance to admit they need help.[1]

Dr. Shlomo Breznitz, an Israeli psychologist, has identified seven types of denial that people use to cope with stress, anxiety, threatening information or uncomfortable emotions. Although his work applies to smoking, we can relate the stages of denial to emotional eating disorders as well:

Stage 1. Denial of Personal Relevance. "I heard bulimia can be dangerous, but I don't throw up enough to cause myself any health problems. I'm not that bad."

Stage 2. Denial of Urgency. "I may be obese with high blood pressure, but there's plenty of time to lose weight when I get around to it."

Stage 3. Denial of Vulnerability. "Plenty of girls are anorexic. Just look at all the pro-anorexia web sites on the internet. No big deal."

Stage 4. Denial of Feelings. "I know I should do something about my laxative use sooner or later, but I'm not really worried."

Stage 5. Denial of Source of Feelings. "Just because I don't eat anything during the day has nothing to do with my trouble concentrating in school."

Stage 6. Denial of Threatening Information. "They say throwing up is supposed to erode my teeth? Whatever."

Stage 7. Denial of All Information. "I lost a lot of weight and don't get my period anymore, but I'm fine. People criticize me for being skinny just because they're jealous. Plenty of girls I know are much worse off."

As you begin breaking through your denial, it is important to recognize there is nothing shameful in being resistant to change. Some people become partially ready. Maybe you would like to stop bingeing, but don't know if you want to give up purging. Maybe you want to stop eating so restrictively, but don't want to gain more than three pounds. It is just fine to start the process wherever *you* are. Readiness comes in many stages. At all different stages of readiness, you can create opportunities to get better. Recovery is a process.

Linda, who battled binge eating, described an angel perched on one shoulder and a devil on her other shoulder.

"I cannot get the devil's voice to stop telling me to binge. How do I just get rid of him once and for all?" she demanded.

I responded, "Let's not get rid of him so fast! Let's invite him to the debate and hear him out. That devil may help us learn some important information about why you feel so stuck."

Food for Thought: Breaking through Denial

- Which of your eating disorder behaviors do you want to change?
- What do you not want to change? Or not change just yet?
- Are you actively working on changing any parts of your eating problem?
- Do you want to get better for yourself or for someone else?
- What problems in your life does emotional eating help you to avoid or to "solve?"
- What would you need to learn in order to let go of your addictive behavior with food?
- What "benefits" or pay-offs are you getting from emotional eating?
- What alternative ways to manage stress can you create for yourself? The more varied the repertoire, the more options you have to turn to.

- Write a letter from your inner angel who wants to change and your inner devil who does not. Give them full freedom of expression.

The dilemma of to change or not to change is active in all of us. Understanding our resistance can help clear the pathways so we can move from obstacles toward opportunities to recovery.

As Janice quipped, "I'm weary of my eating struggles, but I'm wary of changing. Now I'm working on willingness to commit. I'm trying to move from weary to wary to willing!

Ambivalence

If only recovery from an eating disorder were straightforward, like recovery from pneumonia. If we take our antibiotics and get plenty of rest, then, with time, we are cured. If only curing eating disorders were that direct and simple.

Often, what stops a person from healing an eating disorder is an inner hesitancy, fear, or ambivalence about wanting to be cured. Here are some clinical examples illustrating why many people develop an understandable attachment to their eating problem and do not want to let go.

Karen: "I am one of eight kids. Only when I became anorexic did my family really give me a lot of attention and concern for the first time. Do I really want to give that up? Maybe their attention is what I'm really hungry for."

Sandy: "All my life, my mother has been depressed and I've had to take care of her. I've always been vigilant to make sure she's OK and not lonely. When she discovered I was throwing up, she really came out of her shell and began to take care of *me*. She had never seemed that worried about me before. I'm guilty to admit that I secretly love how our roles are now reversed—that I am the child and she is the mother for the first time. My bulimia is like a secret gift helping to bring this about."

Charlie: "On my freshman college break at home, my parents realized that I binge at night and sleep all day, and they got worried about my living away from home. They told me that if I didn't stop overeating out of control, they wouldn't let me go back to college. I'm secretly scared of college anyway. I don't know if I can keep up with the other kids or make friends. Maybe I really don't want to go back. This bingeing could give me the perfect excuse."

Obsession with eating—whether it is compulsive eating, bulimia, or anorexia—often deflects a deeper pain. Karen, Sandy, and Charlie want to recover and feel better about themselves on one hand, but they also realize their eating disorder serves a helpful purpose in their lives, a way of handling the anxieties of daily living and a way of avoiding pain.

People often develop an attachment to their eating problem because it is a security blanket, a friend, a companion, comfort, distraction, obsession, and even an identity. Food, after all, is the most available, socially sanctioned, cheapest, mood-altering drug on the market.

Ambivalence about recovery can manifest itself not just as an inner conflict within oneself but as a conflict in communicating with another person. When Jillian wanted to take an extra sandwich in the car for a trip upstate to visit her parents, her boyfriend poked fun at her. "We just ate an hour ago. Why can't you wait, and we'll eat when we get there?" Jake laughed. Jillian had recently discovered that she needed to eat every three to four hours to prevent getting overly hungry, which then often led to bingeing. That structure gave her security. She felt ashamed by Jake's words, so she became ambivalent about whether to stand up for herself and risk his teasing or retreat and abandon her needs. She felt conflicted and weighed the pros and cons. If she gave in to her shame, she might get hungry and later resort to overeating behind Jake's back; if she declared she was going to buy the sandwich and take care of herself, she risked her boyfriend's ridicule. Jillian decided the best technique was not to be defensive but to tell Jake the truth in an unapologetic manner. He then better understood there was a valid reason for her request. The key to her successful communication? Not apologizing for her needs.

It is only natural to be of two minds as you begin to mend from emotional eating. The head wants one thing, the appetites want something else. The road to recovery from an eating disorder is filled with peaks and valleys, pebbles, boulders, plateaus, and stepping-stones. It is a process that ebbs and flows—two steps forward, one step back.

Food for Thought:
Seeking Therapy to Resolve Your Ambivalence

If you continue to have difficulty with mixed feelings about your recovery, psychotherapy can be a vital tool to get unstuck.

The key is finding a therapist who is attuned and respectful of your own degree of readiness to change. Unfortunately, this is not always the case. Cindy had previously attended therapy to end her binge eating. The therapist diagnosed Cindy as a food addict who should completely avoid all foods with white flour and sugar. The therapist also diagnosed that Cindy was addicted to buying shoes, and he required her to make a commitment not to buy any more shoes.

This approach was doomed to fail because the therapist did not work in collaboration with Cindy to get to the root cause of her bingeing and shopping. Nor did he help her strategize alternative behaviors. The therapist's totalitarian manner of restricting Cindy's behavior with food and shoes did not help her to understand the tug of war going on inside of her.

Although Cindy very much wanted her therapist's approval and tried to follow his recommendations, she finally left that treatment feeling defeated and full of self-blame. A therapist's sledgehammer approach will not help people make peace with their fear and ambivalence.

A more compassionate and wise therapist would have validated Cindy's mixed feelings and coaxed her feelings out into the clear light of day. From there, the therapist and Cindy could explore alternative ways to help Cindy feel better about herself without the crutch of a destructive eating disorder or the comfort of shopping. This attitude could rekindle hope in Cindy that progress is possible.

Several other patients have reported frustration with previous treatment experiences when their therapists have asked them to sign a written contract stating, "I will no longer make myself throw up" or "I agree not to use laxatives." These "vows" will be short-lived if your insides are still conflicted and not fully on board. In a similar vein, a therapist who wrote a handbook on anorexia and bulimia states, "One of the things I ask of my patients is to give me their ultimate trust." But trust can never be demanded. It only comes the old-fashioned way: It must be earned over time!

Sometimes psychotherapists mistakenly become cheerleaders who cajole a patient to get better without appreciating the person's underlying conflicts of anxiety and ambivalence. Every person's eating problem requires an approach that meshes with his or her individual needs and degree of readiness to change.

Fear of Success

In addition to issues of motivation, ambivalence, and denial, another impediment to moving forward with healing an eating problem is the fear of success.[2]

Are you afraid to lose weight? If you are bulimic, do you feel a tug to return to throwing up again, even after you have stopped? When you get your eating under control, do you find yourself sabotaging your success?

With almost every patient I have treated for anorexia, bulimia, or compulsive overeating, I have discovered what I call the Fear-of-Success Syndrome. It raises its head in the course of therapy most often at the point when a person starts to get better and exert some control over his or her eating.

In his paper, "Those Wrecked by Success," Sigmund Freud describes how some people, after attaining a long-cherished wish, may fall ill because they cannot tolerate their wish coming true! Many emotional eaters convince themselves they are striving to resolve their destructive food thoughts and behaviors, but an unconscious part of them remains determined NOT to succeed. They then began to sabotage their progress.

Fears of Change and Loss

Key factors contributing to the Fear-of-Success Syndrome are the fear of change and fear of loss that are roused as we heal our eating problems.

Human beings often experience any change, even change for the better, as a loss. Fears of change and loss come in many forms.

Losing a Sense of Identity

Most emotional eaters spend a substantial amount of their thoughts and energy worrying about eating and weight—what they just ate, what they should have eaten instead, what they will eat tomorrow to make up for it. These thoughts and worries become second nature and provide a sense of identity and security. After all, to a great extent, we are what we think about.

Denise, who began therapy weighing over 300 pounds, had lost 100 pounds the previous year, but had gained it all back and more. She felt helpless, frustrated, and in despair when she came to therapy.

Denise came from a very religious family. When she broke away from their strict religious teachings, her wish to lose weight became her new "religion," but with unexpected results. Even though she lost weight, it brought her no solace. "As I got thinner, I also became depressed," Denise revealed. "I had a feeling of loss that was similar to what I felt when I moved away from my family and the religious beliefs I grew up with. If I couldn't worry about dieting and calories, losing and gaining weight, what would give my life meaning? Telling myself I am fat and ugly has been like a daily mantra for me! What am I going to replace that with? If I give up my obsession with food and weight, I worry about feeling empty inside and without any purpose in life."

This identity crisis also occurs in patients who come for therapy following a dramatic, quick weight loss due to surgery or a fast. Maria had lost 110 pounds following gastric bypass surgery, but found herself bingeing again. She came for help in a state of terror, explaining that at her new thin weight, she no longer knew who she was. "I feel like a stranger in a strange land. I now have to learn how to navigate my body through life at this thinner weight— even how to walk down the street, how much space I need to sit on a bus. It scares me. All of this is so new. I don't even know what style clothes I like or what size I should wear. Even my own face looks unfamiliar."

Both Denise and Maria found themselves in a period of transition and mourning that many emotional eaters experience when their obsession with food is no longer at the front and center of their lives. The ability to tolerate this transition period and work through it is a vital key to sustained recovery.

When you begin to recognize how much your sense of identity has been wrapped up in your eating struggle, you will be more prepared for the onslaught of feelings or backlash that arises as you recover. It takes courage to grow and succeed. Growing pains got its name because sometimes growing hurts!

Losing the Status Quo in Relationships
Sometimes weight and eating disorders play a part in the balance of power, trust, and dependency in relationships. Getting better means having to find new ways of relating to others.

Peter's wife and daughter badgered him constantly about losing weight. In despair, they finally joined a family support group which helped them recognize the futility of trying to control Peter's behavior. As they backed off from monitoring and criticizing him, Peter discovered how much he missed their complaining about his weight! He was shocked to realize how their attention had made him feel cared for and special. He said, "It was similar to my parents, where my mother repeatedly yelled at my father to stop drinking. I never understood that I interpreted her reprimands as a way of showing Dad love and attention. I'm beginning to see my own need to be scolded by my wife and daughter is some kind of misguided attempt to get their affection. But, instead, it is really eroding their respect for me."

Power struggles between husbands and wives about weight can also affect the status quo of their relationship. Imagine the stress and confusion of a wife whose husband says, "Honey, you really need to lose a couple of pounds." But just as Honey starts losing those pounds, he suddenly becomes worried. He fears he is losing his edge to criticize her and be the boss. What does he do? He brings her a box of chocolates to celebrate her weight loss!

Sometimes being successful feels like being disloyal to one's family, and so we sacrifice ourselves to continue to belong. Betsy came from a family of obese parents and two obese brothers who shared an ongoing camaraderie about their weight. When Betsy went away to college, she was able to get more in touch with her own rhythm of eating and lost 20 pounds. But when she returned home for Christmas, her family treated her as if she had deserted them. "Boy, look at her," they said. "College makes you think you're too good for us. We have two weeks to fatten you up again!"

Betsy was devastated by her family's disapproval and began to feel guilty about her change in size. She started to overeat to undo her achievement and return to the family fold. In therapy, though, she realized that regaining the weight was her way of trying to keep the relationship with her family intact. She also understood that her success—whether it was enjoying her body more or achieving a college education—would entail some degree of growing beyond and apart from her family. As she slowly resolved this anxiety and guilt about separating from her family, she was able to get back on track with her new-found patterns of healthier eating.

Losing a Sense of Sexual Protection

Making our bodies either very skinny or very fat is often an attempt to feel more powerful and in control when it comes to sex. Some anorexic girls starve themselves to diminish their feminine curves; anorexic boys seek to lessen their muscular development in the hope of de-sexualizing themselves. Reducing one's body to that of a child is an attempt, in part, to ward off the fears and responsibilities of sexuality.

Others who make their bodies large through bingeing may also be trying to desexualize themselves. "The more space my body takes up, the more distance there is between you and me. To lose that protection can feel dangerous and scary."

Lauren had been sexually abused by her uncle when she was ten. At age 19, she found herself in a sexual situation with a man from work and became terrified. She feared this man would overpower her and she would be left vulnerable, without any control over the situation. She began gaining weight, hoping it would shield her from his advances.

In therapy, Lauren and I worked together to help her relive and resolve the pain of her uncle's abuse. Gradually, she began to separate her past experience from her present. She discovered that she *did* want to connect with this man, but in a manner that felt comfortable for her. Lauren worked on developing the realm of "maybe," which included a degree of flirtation. Lauren didn't necessarily want the four-course meal, but she wanted to try the appetizer—to laugh and banter and be playful. Flirting gave Lauren another option besides retreating. It also enabled her to feel more in control of the contact and less dependent on her weight to protect her. In time, she even felt secure enough to taste the main course!

In truth, becoming skinny or fat does not have the power to desexualize us. People of all sizes and shapes can be sexually active and satisfied. Real power lies in having choices and in developing our ability to express and act on those choices: learning to say yes when we mean yes, learning to say no when we mean no, and learning to say maybe when we haven't quite decided.

Losing Other Women's Approval

Fear of alienating other women and losing their support is an undercurrent for many women who begin to gain healthier bodies and feel more attractive. Being overweight, or even significantly underweight, says to other women: "I am not a threat. You don't have to worry about my being prettier than you or stealing all the attention." Sometimes succeeding in feeling more in harmony with your body brings with it a fear of becoming more competitive with other women.

Envy and competition can be uncomfortable feelings for women. Sometimes, having our girlfriends envy us validates our success, but it also brings with it the possibility they will withdraw their affection and desert us. The question then arises, "How powerful or attractive can I become without causing my friends to reject me?"

In *Between Women,* Luise Eichenbaum and Susie Orbach explain, "We can feel guilty for our strivings and seek punishment for them. The unconscious equation that fulfilling oneself, succeeding in one's career, or achieving a personally satisfying love relationship is a betrayal of another woman (mother) is extremely common. We can imagine or project onto one another disapproval and in this way we hold each other back."[3]

Arthur Miller, in his memoir *Timebends,* discusses the root of his fear of success, an insight that is applicable for emotional eaters: "I was not the first to experience the guilt of success and though I suspected the truth, I was unable to do much about it: such guilt is a protective device to conceal one's happiness at surpassing others, especially those one loves, like a brother, father or friend. It is a kind of payment to them in the form of pseudo remorse. But this is not altogether a phantom exercise, for the psyche knows that those who have been surpassed may harbor thoughts of retaliation that can be dangerous in reality. So one speaks through such guilt—'Don't bother resenting me, I've failed too.' "[4]

This is not a perfect world, and there will always be some who resent our recovery from food and weight obsession. But the more we can tolerate their envy and let the problem be theirs and not ours, the more we will hold onto our successes and not abandon ourselves by returning to emotional eating.

Naomi told her eating support group that whenever she felt more attractive, she became afraid that her girlfriends would not like her anymore. Naomi's mother had been a fashion model and always needed to be the most beautiful woman in the family. The friends Naomi brought home from school often said in surprise, *"That's* your mother?" impressed by Mrs. Fisher's glamour.

When Naomi began blossoming at age 13, her mother became quite critical of her. "I couldn't win," she said. "My mother always needed to be prettier and sexier. There was room for only one attractive female in our house—she made that clear. For me, not bingeing anymore and losing weight brings back awful memories of my mother's competitiveness and makes me think my girlfriends are going to hate me. In my eating support group, though, I'm learning these women are *not* my mother. They applaud my progress. They want me to succeed. This is very healing for me. Enjoying and nurturing my body doesn't have to lead to disapproval or abandonment."

Losing Physical Protection

For some people, changes in body image alter their sense of security in the world. Overweight people, for instance, may fear they will be physically vulnerable at a smaller size and so, subconsciously, they hold onto their fat as protection. Patients in my eating support groups have even expressed uneasiness about losing weight because they associated thinness with the pain of a loved one becoming emaciated from cancer.

Many of my patients were afraid to lose the protection they attributed to their larger bodies.

Ruth: "When I was nine years old, a girl in my class fell between the subway cars and was killed. She had just lost over 50 pounds, and I kept thinking if she were still fat she wouldn't have been able to fall between those cars. This made an enormous impression on me, and I started to link my own weight loss with the fear that something terrible could happen to me, too."

Annette: "I was hit by a bicycle last week, and I remember thinking, 'It's a good thing I'm fat or I would have gotten really hurt.' "

Lois: "My father was fat all his life, and in the last two years the doctors convinced him to lose weight because his health was in jeopardy. He finally did lose 65 pounds, but died six months later from a stroke. I always believed that if he hadn't lost so much weight, he never would have died. It made me scared that could happen to me."

As irrational as these thoughts may seem, they nevertheless can exert a powerful influence on our willingness to make peace with food and allow our bodies to reach their natural weight. These connections need to be uncovered and untangled so their power can be lessened.

Losing the Power to Spite Someone

From the minute she was born, it seemed to Alice that her mother only wanted two things from her: that she be slim and get married to someone rich. But try as she might, Alice could not lose the extra

50 pounds her mother hated and only managed to meet unsuitable guys. "Since I was a little girl, my mother measured out my food and weighed me weekly. I hated scales. I hated measuring cups. I hated her! Whenever her back was turned, I would sneak candy and cookies. Staying fat was perfect revenge and, even though I'm now 25, my mother is still trying to control my weight and marital status—and I'm still reacting!

"What's pathetic about my story," Alice continued, "is that I'd really like to have normal eating habits and get married some day. But another part of me enjoys getting back at her more than getting my life together. I'm in such a bind!"

Alice knew that if she did lose weight, she would also lose a powerful weapon of spite against her mother. Staying large is her way of communicating, "I'm going to be my own person, and you can't do anything about it!" This is reminiscent of the daughter in the movie, *Summer Wishes, Winter Dreams,* who yells at her mother, "Don't criticize me about my weight. It's the only thing that's mine, and you are not going to take that away from me!"

Only when Alice learns to separate her wishes and hopes for herself from the coercion and pressure she experiences from her mother will she permit herself to attain her natural weight. This means asserting herself directly, rather than letting her body do the talking for her. Then, her decisions will come from within *her* and not from her mother. As a colleague of mine once said, "Maturity is doing something *even though* your mother wants it!"

Food for Thought: How to Be Your Own Therapist

If your obsession with food and weight were solved, what would you replace it with? What would you be thinking about instead? Would you miss it?

- Since when has your eating disorder been a coping mechanism for you? Why did it start then?
- When people say you look like you lost weight, does that trigger anxiety? Does it provoke renewed eating problems?
- When you start eating more healthfully, do you ever feel more emotional and vulnerable—more anger, depression, anxiety, loneliness?
- Do you worry that resolving your eating problem might cause upset in an important relationship in your life?
- When you begin to get on track with your eating, do you sabotage your progress, often without realizing it?
- What about giving up emotional eating are you *really* afraid of? What's *really* holding you back?

If you were living in harmony with your body and expressing your feelings without detouring them through dieting, bingeing, purging or starving:

- How would your family life change? Your work life? Your friendships?
- In what ways would these changes be negative or frightening?
- In what ways would these changes be positive or exhilarating?
- Are there any other dangers about declaring peace with your food and eating that could get in your way?

In *Necessary Losses*, Judith Viorst reminds us that losses are a necessary and vital part of life that can spur us on to change and grow. She writes, "The road to human development is paved with renunciation. Throughout our life we grow by giving up. We give up some of our deepest attachments to others. We give up certain cherished parts of ourselves. We must confront all that we will never have and never will be. We grow by losing and leaving and letting go. We grow by changing and moving on."[5]

1   Shlomo Breznitz, *Maximum Brainpower: Challenging the Brain for Health and Wisdom* (Ballantine Books, 2012).

2   Mary Anne Cohen, *French Toast for Breakfast: Declaring Peace with Emotional Eating.* (Gürze Books, 1995). Material on the fear of success has been adapted from this book.

3   Luise Eichenbaum and Susie Orbach, *Between Women* (Penguin Books, 1987).

4   Arthur Miller, *Timebends: A Life* (Penguin Books, 1995), 139.

5   Judith Viorst, *Necessary Losses* (Simon & Schuster, 1986).

9. Psychotherapy: A Second Chance

In the deserts of the heart
Let the healing fountains start.

—W.H. Auden

Psychotherapy is a healing conversation that provides an opportunity to repair the wounds of childhood and insecure attachment.[1] The relationship with the therapist can help mend the patient's mistrust and inner rage.

Stuart was a 44-year-old man with a history of job difficulties, few friends, and bulimia. In his therapy, a frequent topic was his considerable resentment of others and how bingeing and purging became his solution to rid himself of chronic pent-up anger.

Stuart arrived at my office one warm summer's day and became annoyed at me for not having turned on the air conditioning. "It's so hot in here. Don't you give a damn about anyone but yourself?" he snarled. "I know what your problem is. You're a cheap bastard! You're such a cheap bastard you probably want to charge your clients extra for the air conditioning. And how about the toilet paper—do you want to charge extra for that as well?" he sneered.

Of all the names I may have been called in my life, "cheap bastard" is not one of them. I recognized that Stuart was casting me in the role of someone from his past. He continued to yell at me about my fee, my cancellation policy, the tiresome stairs to my office, and other indications of what he considered my selfishness. "I hate you," he yelled. "I hate you. I hate you! You are just like my father—a mean, selfish bastard. We were eight children growing up and he never put in air conditioning for us. Every summer after sweltering summer our house was like an oven. Pop had the money, but he didn't care about us. When it came time to sell the house, guess what? He installed *central* air so he'd get a better price!"

Stuart's relationship with me triggered an explosion of bitterness that stemmed from his father's not valuing him or taking him into consideration. In casting me as the selfish father, he connected with his strong emotional deprivation. His past became alive in the present, where he was now able to vent his rage and bring it out into the clear light of day.

As Stuart realized I would not retaliate against him, he poured out toxic feelings of fury to me and to his father for failing to make him feel important. He began to use his mouth to express his hostility, instead of resorting to bingeing and puking. Having a channel to express himself directly with me gave him options far more gratifying than his eating disorder.

When the therapist becomes the "bad guy," it often means important work is emerging. Once the patient feels safe to unleash his anger and reflects on its meaning, the treatment takes hold in an enriched way. Eventually, as in the case of Stuart, he comes to realize the therapist is not a cheap bastard like the father. He becomes aware he has seen the world through a lens of deprivation, and begins to reassess more realistically his current relationships with the world.

In *Roadblocks on the Journey of Psychotherapy*, Jane Hall explains, "The therapist and the patient are two real human beings who develop a unique relationship but most of the script in the drama was written in the past. As it is played out in the present, the therapist's interpretations invite the patient to revise the script based on new experiences." When old difficulties too painful to resolve reemerge with the therapist, the patient has a second chance to work through troubling familiar scenarios and begins to resolve them. The therapist becomes a new attachment figure modeling acceptance, compassion, understanding, reflection.[2]

Stuart perceived over time that I understood and empathized with his feelings. This was a far cry from his father's reply to his complaints, "Just get over yourself. You kids have it a hell of a lot better than I ever did!" These retorts always made Stuart feel guilty, unlovable, and even more enraged. My acceptance and validation of his feelings led him to believe he was entitled to feel sympathy for himself.

The nurturing relationship with the therapist provides healing because it repairs the core of the patient's wounded relationships. The therapist works with the patient to understand his or her early attachment history and also helps the patient understand how that history relates to the present difficulties. By integrating both the past and the present, the therapist and the patient create an individualized treatment approach. Emotional eaters develop the capacity to regulate their emotions, not act on impulsive feelings, tolerate discomfort, reflect on the meaning of their emotions, turn to others for security, and learn to love. These are the tasks of creating a healthy and integrated self.

However, many people dislike the idea of developing a strong relationship with the therapist or becoming dependent on a therapist. They say, "I just want to get fixed from my eating disorder," or "I don't want a relationship with you," or "Just let me get on with my life." They often pose pointed questions to the therapist that reveal their personal fears about the treatment process, as well as relationships in general:

- What if you become a crutch to me, just like the food?
- What if I need you more than you need me, which I assume must be the case?
- How can you really care for me if this is just a business to you and I pay you?
- I feel like a fool revealing all my inner insecurities and I know nothing about you. It doesn't feel fair.
- You have so many other patients. Do you feel the same way about everyone?
- What if I get close to you and never want to leave therapy?
- How will I know when I'm ready to leave? Will you let me leave? After all, you'll be losing the money you get from me.
- My last therapist died during my therapy. How do I know the same thing won't happen here with you?
- How do you remember what I say? Do you write down notes about me?
- What if I say something that hurts your feelings and you don't like me anymore? Will you pretend to help me but instead lead me on the wrong path out of spite?
- What if I have sexual feelings to you?
- Do you ever have sexual feelings for your patients?
- Do you ever pretend to care when you really don't?
- Will you think about me when you're on vacation or do you forget all about your patients when you're out of the office? Will you miss me?
- Did you know that the word "therapist" is actually "the-rapist?"
- Did you ever lie to a client? Would you ever lie to me?
- If I get better, will you take all the credit?
- Do you love me?

Obviously, these questions are laden with meaning that a mere yes or no can't answer. The therapist's stock answer, which has been turned into a joke that pokes fun at shrinks, is "What do you mean by that?" This question often leaves people feeling rebuffed and patronized. However, the therapist's *intention* in asking, "What do you mean by that?" is valid—to discover and explore the unique thoughts and ideas of each person.

If, for example, a woman asks me, "Do you ever have sexual feelings for your patients?" and she is someone who has been the victim of sexual abuse, then I surmise she is trying to determine if I can be trusted not to act out sexually or impulsively. But the question could mean she is struggling with her own homosexual feelings to me; or it could mean she wants to be mothered intimately like a little girl. A sensitive therapist will help patients identify their specific concerns.

If a young teenage boy poses the same question, he may wonder what kinds of sexual feelings are acceptable and normal. I may kid him and say, "Is the idea of my having sexual feelings to you something you fear or you wish?" or "What would it feel like if I did?" or "Is there something specific you would like to do with me?"

Caring therapists believe every client question has meaning that needs to be deciphered and every question has value. Therapists need to respect their patients' inquiries, as uncomfortable as they may be. When clients ask difficult and intrusive questions, it may also be their way of turning the tables on the therapist and putting the therapist in the hot seat.

Emotional eaters have subsumed their inner lives behind struggles with food and weight. The emotional eater's world has narrowed into the world of numbers: How can I lose 20 pounds quickly? How can I get back to wearing a size 6? I'll just have an apple for lunch—it's only 100 calories.

They are fluent in the language of eating disorders, but not so much in the language of feelings and self-expression. Questions to the therapist can deepen the treatment into richer, more alive concerns. The curiosity of the therapist and the therapist's own genuine personal involvement foster the growing self-reflection of the patient. Rather than taking an action (like overeating), patients are encouraged to wonder about their feelings, their reactions, their behavior. This work will finally help the person claim her true and vital appetite for life!

Bodies Come Alive in Therapy

In the therapy session, we are more than just two minds and two hearts. The intimacy between patient and therapist extends beyond verbal communication. We are also two bodies. Patients have emotional reactions to the therapist's body which, when deciphered, can help illuminate issues of body image, envy, hate, sexuality. Especially in the therapy of eating disorders, where concerns about size, shape, weight, and appearance are so paramount, reactions to the therapist's body are often a valuable topic to be discussed and understood. My hair style, my gray hair, my breasts, my weight, my eyes, my jewelry, my clothes, my sexual orientation, my hay fever sneezing have all been commented on by patients at different times. One patient even asked me if I ever suffered from explosive diarrhea like she had!

Not only do patients observe me and my body, but I also observe how the patients who sit before me speak to me in body language. I have had many nursing mothers proudly uncover their breasts to feed their babies in my office; a vegetarian patient with chronic garlic breath that smelled up the whole room; a teenager who displayed ample cleavage and hiked up her skirt in sessions; a patient whose little daughter climbed on my lap cuddling with me in session and gave me a case of head lice; and a man who tracked mud into my bathroom, leaving it for me to clean up.

In session, tears spill, noses are runny, sweaty bodies exude their odor, farts occasionally ring out, perfume may sweeten the office as does the aura of cigarette or cigar smoke—these are the earthy components of the therapy relationship. The patient who may feel inadequate, like a nobody (she has "no body" that she loves) is witnessed in her bodily humanity and accepted without judgment by the therapist.

They are also sending me a message. A nonverbal message. A body language message that needs to be translated into words as patient and therapist work together.[3]

All of these nonverbal communications are intimate expressions of attachment. The therapist's body and the patient's body speak. The connection is deepened; the attachment comes alive; hope takes root.

The therapist moves the patient from the language of the body to expressive language by creating a "verbal bridge" which is "like a hand extended to the patient, inviting her to cross over" to help her satisfy the craving to feel that she is "living full, warm, and juicy in her own skin."[4]

The Eating Disorder Mirrors the Therapy Relationship

To the surprise of patients, the relationship they develop with their therapist will often begin to parallel the relationship they have with food. This connection with the therapist then becomes a mirror to better understand their inner world of emotional eating, providing a rich avenue of exploration.[5]

The eating styles of the anorexic, the compulsive eater, and the bulimic reflect the kind of relationship each develops with the people in their lives.

The Therapy Relationship and the Anorexic

The root of the anorexic disorder, in which the person prides herself on avoiding food and denying hunger, is directly related to the person's early family relationships.

Jody was a tiny, sparrow-like girl who had been anorexic since age 12. She described how her father held court at the dinner table each night, lecturing his children, lecturing his wife, raising his voice, and intimidating his family. Jody's stomach would close up with tension at these times, but her father forbade anyone to leave the table until they cleaned their plate. Usually, she forced herself to finish by choking down her food.

This was only one of many painful memories Jody had of her father's domination over the family. Now in her early 20s, she led a restricted life with few close friends and also greatly feared her boss at work. Although she appeared emaciated, Jody came to therapy not to be helped for anorexia, but for the deep loneliness and emptiness she felt inside.

Whenever I offered support and understanding to her in our session, Jody withdrew from me. It was as if my words made her wince. Then I realized that she experienced my words, like her father's, as being *forced* down her throat. She felt obligated to "swallow" my interpretations. But how could I help her if I couldn't verbally communicate?

I began experimenting with silence and discovered that the less I talked, the more Jody slowly came alive. Because her experience had been that her body, mind, and soul were the possessions of her father, to receive an interpretation from me was to confirm her sense of inadequacy, as if I, too, were telling her what to think and feel. But when I became more passive, Jody emerged to take the reins of the sessions rather than feeling "force fed" by me. As she came to control more of the therapy space we shared, Jody also began eating more. Finally, feeling more in control of both her eating and her relationships, she was slowly able to let go of her need to fend off food and relationships with people.

The Therapy Relationship and the Compulsive Eater

Compulsive eaters relate to their therapists in a variety of ways. Many feel they cannot "get enough" from the therapist. They demand, "Tell me what to do. Give me advice. Talk to me." Feeling deprived, they turn to food and to the therapist to fill up the empty place inside. Some complain that their previous therapists did not talk enough, leaving them feeling cheated and hungry for more. Obviously, my role as therapist in this case is not to fill up my patient by talking incessantly but to tune in when she is feeling emotionally hungry and try to understand what is triggering her feelings of emptiness at that moment.

Other patients work hard at guarding *against* their hungry inner self in order not to burden the therapist too much. I know I am sitting with this kind of "defensive" overeater when I start feeling bored or sleepy. My own boredom alerts me that my patient is struggling to keep her distance from her own emotions and from me. She relates intellectually, as if reciting an essay entitled, "My Emotional Problems," which is her way of protecting us both from what she believes is her unbearable, repulsive neediness.

This was the case of Janet, an obese 33-year-old gay woman who had been a compulsive eater since childhood. Shortly after she was born, her mother became ill, and Janet was sent to live with her grandmother. Then, when she was five, her mother began having outbursts of rage, pulling Janet's hair and hitting her with a wooden spoon.

It was revealed in therapy that Janet had come to believe she was bad for needing and wanting too much and that her voracious appetite for care and attention had driven her mother away. Overeating became a disguise and diverted her from her real need for sustenance from others.

In Janet's eyes, I quickly became Ms. Perfect Therapist. I could do no wrong. Janet would pull her chair up close to mine in my office and scrutinize my face attentively. As we got to know each other better, she revealed how she searched my face to determine whether or not I was angry at her. Just as she had feared her mother's random and unexplained explosions, she now feared mine. And even though we kept working on Janet's overeating and bingeing, she found little relief.

Then, after my summer vacation, which came at a difficult time for Janet because her grandmother was dying, I began feeling in our sessions together that she wanted to bite me, both to extract more emotional milk/nourishment and to express her anger that I was not there when she needed me. Evidently my vacation had brought up old bruises and feelings of abandonment, but Janet was too afraid to reveal her anger toward me. She continued biting into food instead of "biting" me.

Following a particularly needy session in which she was upset about her grandmother's illness, she asked, "When will you be taking your next vacation? I think you should take one soon."

"What makes you ask about my vacation at this point?" I inquired.

"You look tired and probably need some time away from your patients," she said.

I said, "You feel that your neediness drains me, and you are sucking me dry . . ."

She interrupted, "I feel I want so much from you that you should go away and restore yourself."

"You seem to believe I have a finite amount to give you and that you may use it all up," I continued. "You are scared of wanting too much from me—that I will get angry with you and pull away from you."

Although she continued to be fearful of her voracious feelings, a gradual shift occurred in our work together after this session. Instead of constantly asking, "Is our time over yet?" which meant "I am afraid I have been a bad girl and taken too much from you," Janet began to ask, "Do we have some more time left?" I understood her rephrasing the question to mean, "I am able to admit that I have hungry needs and I want more from you. Maybe I'm not so bad to admit that I want more."

As Janet gradually took in my soothing presence and realized I accepted her even when she was angry and hungry, she was able to interrupt her own binge with new-found coping methods. She began turning more to her friends and me rather than gorging on food.

The Therapy Relationship and the Bulimic

The bingeing and purging pattern of the bulimic also parallels her style of relating to people. She will let herself get close to someone, only to eventually reject and dismiss them, banishing the relationship from her system just as she does the food. A most astonishing example of this occurred in my initial evaluation with Gladys, who informed me over the phone that she had been bingeing and vomiting for the past 13 years.

From the first moment we met, Gladys disliked me. She said I looked like her last therapist, Ms. Morgan, who had abandoned her practice to join a cult religion. Ms. Morgan had written a letter to Gladys saying her job on the commune was to scrub toilets, and she felt uplifted in a way she never had as a therapist! Gladys had decided on first viewing that I could not be trusted—just as her bulimic self had decided many years before that food could not be trusted. Reassurance that I would not abandon her abruptly nor leave her to scrub toilets (I barely had time to tend my own!) would have fallen on deaf ears.

Gladys told me she could not trust me nor did she want to work with me. "But I do not expect you to trust me," I said. Some of her other therapists had tried to convince her they were indeed trustworthy, while I recognized that Gladys' "not trusting" position was exactly where she needed to be at the beginning of our relationship.

So we began on this rocky road. As Gladys's therapy unfolded, she confided what life had been like for her when she was growing up. She had adored her handsome father and always turned to him for comfort when she was little, even though he drank too much. But when she was six, as she lay cuddled in his arms, he began to fondle her sexually, stroking and rubbing her body.

Gladys' world shattered to pieces. Her father's betrayal had destroyed forever her innocence and trust. He had turned on her and had become poison, just as later in life, food—the comforting nurturer—would become poison as well. This mistrust of her father not only spilled over to food but to all her relationships as well. Now, her suspicions became reflected in her relationship with me, her therapist.

For this reason, our relationship became *the* avenue to discover and explore Gladys's inner world. Every time she wanted to leave therapy and "spit me out," we worked on tracing back what had triggered this new episode of mistrust with me. For the first time, she was able to express her wariness without worrying that I would be angry or retaliate. This translated into her ability to trust her food as well, and hold it down. Understanding these parallels between her early life, her food, and her apprehensions also gave Gladys a sense of relief that she wasn't crazy—her behavior had rhyme and reason.

Just as the disappointments we experience with the people we love became the original reason we turn to emotional eating, so must nourishing human relationships become the path toward our cure. The courage to turn to a therapist to unravel one's problems is a crucial step in undoing the bond with food and replacing it with human nurturing.

Emotional eating has frozen our feelings and pains. The relationship with the therapist can help us thaw.

1   The phrase psychotherapy is "a healing conversation" is attributed to Andrea Levin, LCSW.

2   Jane Hall, *Roadblocks on the Journey of Psychotherapy* (Jason Aronson, 2004), 175, 187, 258.

3   It seems to me that one of the downsides to therapy sessions by telephone or Skype is these vivid body communications are never captured.

4   Sharon Farber, *When the Body Is the Target: Self-Harm, Pain, and Traumatic Attachments* (Jason Aaronson, 2002).

5   Adapted from Mary Anne Cohen, *French Toast for Breakfast* (Gürze Books, 1995), 171–177.

10. Food, Glorious Food! Declaring Peace with Emotional Eating

Judith called the New York Center for Eating Disorders in despair. "I'm out of control with my eating. I need to get back in control. Can I come in to see you?"

Judith came prepared with a series of questions about how the process of treatment for emotional eating works.

To get a behind-the-scenes look at psychotherapy for emotional eating, let's use Judith's questions as a launching pad to describe the process.

What Is Therapy for Emotional Eating?

Psychotherapy helps people discover the connection between the emotional stress in their lives and their eating problems. A person under emotional strain may turn to food for comfort by bingeing, or by purging her food for relief of tension if she is bulimic, or by starving herself to gain a sense of control if she is anorexic. Each person has his or her own unique emotional trigger points, such as anxiety, anger, depression, resentment, sadness at a loss, grief over the death of a loved one, loneliness, boredom, rejection, frustration.

The first step is for the person to describe the history of how and when her eating problem began and the impact her eating issues have had on her life. She recounts the emotional worries she is dealing with, what steps she has taken to help herself, and who are the important people in her life. The goal from the outset is to help the person explore the connection between her emotions and her eating and then find alternatives. This is why therapy is sometimes called "the talking cure."

The therapist is an emotional companion on the journey toward healing an eating disorder. The root of the word "companion" comes from the Latin and means "to break bread." *(com* = with, *pan* = bread). To break bread is an act of sharing, of togetherness, of comfort, of being present in the moment.

In the initial stage of therapy, patients are often relieved to learn that turning to food for comfort can stem from a *healthy* impulse. It is a simple, direct, and honest attempt to make oneself feel better immediately in order to better cope with anxiety. Food, after all, is the cheapest, most available, legal, and socially sanctioned mood-altering substance around. The problem is, in the long run, using food to try to solve life's problems backfires. The person is left feeling empty, unfulfilled, and unhappy with her body. And the original issues that prompted the person to seek solace in food have not gotten resolved.

In the early stages of therapy, I work to develop specific "non-food nurturing" strategies for clients to soothe and comfort themselves without unwanted eating behavior. We devise alternatives each person can use to feel better without recruiting bingeing, purging, or starving. It may mean something as simple as taking a nap, or listening to music, taking a shower, taking a walk, writing in a diary, or even having a meal. To break through the solitary confinement of emotional eating may mean replacing isolation with pastry with intimacy with people.

The objective is twofold: to become aware of the emotional triggers that set the unwanted behavior in motion and, at the same time, to relieve the eating disorders symptoms through behavioral changes.

Awareness must be coupled with behavioral change. Neither is sufficient to sustain ongoing relief and recovery from emotional eating. I believe that:

$$\text{Awareness} + \text{Action} = \text{Results}$$

Why Therapy?

Attending a weight-loss program or consulting with a nutritionist are fine resources a person can use in her quest to resolve her eating problems. I often refer people to these support services. Weight-loss programs can be helpful by providing a structure, a format to organize one's food, and a community of people to share with. A nutritionist can also help by custom-tailoring a personal food plan that takes into account whatever health issues you may have, such as high cholesterol, heart disease, diabetes, or prediabetes.

However, if you have struggled with eating problems for many years, it may mean you have not resolved the emotional strains that fuel your eating disorder. All the structured eating plans or nutritional advice in the world will only last for a short time if those other forces are operating within you, calling you back to the food.

Judith, for instance, believed that if she only lost weight, her self-image problems would be solved. But no matter what diet or weight loss program she tried, she was only "good" for a brief period.

What emerged in Judith's therapy was that she was depressed in her marriage. She often felt belittled by her husband or ignored by his heavy work demands. Left alone with little support, Judith suppressed her anger and overate at night as a way of compensating for not feeling loved and respected. Therapy helped Judith face her resentment and how she used overeating to stifle and squash her anger. She realized she needed to speak up more directly to her husband about these dissatisfactions, or they were never going to get better. Judith had never previously made the connection between her nighttime binges and her stifled anger.

Did making this connection help her eating? The answer is yes and no. Rather than running mindlessly to the refrigerator, Judith began asking herself instead what she was feeling en route to the kitchen. Sometimes, this gave her a chance to stop in her tracks and think about what was bothering her and how to better handle it without the food. Other times, she had no idea what else to do and kept her rendezvous with the ice cream. And then, increasingly, instead of using her mouth for eating, she went back to the living room and used her mouth for speaking. She confronted her husband about her dismay at his ignoring her. Over time, Judith and her husband began to improve this issue together.

The point of Judith's story is that change does not happen all at once. Improvements—especially long-lasting ones—take time and patience. As she developed greater self-awareness and more reflection about the feelings that sparked her eating, Judith was able, little by little, to put a stop to her compulsive eating and eat more mindfully.

What Goes on in Therapy for Emotional Easting?

Sometimes we spend the session talking about a person's week with food—what went right, what was not so great. We try to understand the patterns and trigger points that provoke emotional eating, and then we plot what to do next. Sometimes people keep a food and mood journal to help us get a better perspective of their week with food. This often highlights what situations, people, or places can provoke eating problems.

Sometimes the topic of food never even comes up in a therapy session. *This does not mean that you are not actively working on your eating problem.* It means that you are bringing up other meaningful issues that have affected your eating and stress levels.

As we saw with Judith, an eating disorder is about food and *not* about food at the same time. People with eating disorders enlist food to soothe and distract themselves from deep and sometimes upsetting feelings. In each session, we look at the unique interplay between food and emotions.

Clients may revert to hurtful eating behaviors even after they have made some progress. After all, it can be scary to lose weight, or to stop purging if you are bulimic, or to stop starving if you are anorexic. These abuses of food may have been your way of managing feelings for years. As you begin to make progress with your eating disorder, self-ambushes may sabotage success. Often a hidden fear of success is rooted in one's heart. This is where psychotherapy is valuable. No amount of Weight Watchers or nutrition counseling—as helpful and beneficial as they may be—will resolve this kind of ingrained issue.

Will I Lose Weight in Therapy for Emotional Easting?

Maybe. When you no longer use food as a reaction to inner tension, you will begin to reconnect your eating with *physical* hunger, not emotional hunger. The key is to eat because of hunger in the stomach and not hunger from the heart.

Eventually you will arrive at your set-point, the weight range that your body was naturally meant to be. If you are committed to a size 4 when your natural body type and genetics dictate a size 16, you will be disappointed. You have a choice. You can redouble your exercise and food restrictions (which most times results in a backlash of over-eating). Or, you can bemoan your fate and hate the way you look for the rest of your life. Or, you can try to understand why you are wedded to achieving a weight that is clearly not in harmony with your heredity.

Making peace with the weight that nature intended for you can be a challenge, since we live in a culture where appearance and image are highly emphasized. Many women often flounder at this point in their recovery because of the ingrained notion that the thinner they are, the better and "hotter" they are. This dooms them to a life of perpetual dissatisfaction and needs to be worked out in their therapy. Self-acceptance takes time to achieve, but it is worth the effort, because you are going to have to live with yourself for the rest of your life!

Judith was able to lose some weight following a strategy of not swallowing her feelings. Other people learn to improve their habits and become healthier but do not necessarily lose all the weight they desire. We know how heredity and metabolism can set the point of one's natural weight. There is no guarantee you will lose all the weight you want in emotional eating therapy. However, your eating patterns will improve, your capacity to deal with stress will improve, and you will resolve issues from the past that were self-destructive and caused you unhappiness.

Dr. William Davis of the Renfrew Center, a leading eating disorders treatment center, adds this insight: "Dealing with weight itself is not the point. Instead . . . weight change *may* be a byproduct of learning to listen to oneself and care for oneself in a new, more accepting and more *wholesome* way. Healing occurs when someone comes to value knowing, nourishing, respecting and guiding *all* of herself. In this circumstance, physical health and emotional health are joined in a positive, life-affirming manner."[1]

How Long Will Therapy Take?

Unless your problem just began last month, recovery is a process that takes time and patience. We saw in Judith's case that after she experienced many layers of self-realization over time, she healed her eating problem.

After four sessions of psychotherapy, Peggy's husband did not notice any great change in Peggy's overeating habits. As a successful businessman, he was used to quick, concrete results in his business. He wanted to know why she was not cured yet. His pressure made Peggy ashamed that she wasn't working fast enough in her therapy. Peggy was convinced that her only problem in life was that she was too fat. If she could only lose weight, she thought, she would be fine. Since she wasn't losing weight in therapy fast enough, she was ready to give up.

I pointed out to Peggy that she was in mourning for her sister who had recently died, she was in the process of buying a new house, and she had a long history of binge eating dating back to her teenage years. Peggy underestimated how all these tensions in her life were causing a resurgence of her eating disorder. She needed time to calm down, appreciate, and "digest" the losses and challenges she was undergoing. Peggy also needed to learn that eating disorders are often a person's attempt to distract herself from the grieving process. When she became aware of this, she decided to take the time she needed to fully sort through her problems without feeling like a failure. Peggy's overeating ebbed as she felt better understood.

The process of therapy is a journey of collaboration and exploration that does not occur overnight. With self-reflection and self-compassion, patience and perseverance, you can declare peace with emotional eating.

You can learn to sink your teeth into life, not into excess food!

Food Rehabilitation

"I'm trying to lose weight, and I got these low-calorie crackers. They taste like a mixture of cardboard and sawdust, but at least they don't have many calories and they do fill me up!" Bruce described.

Bruce's description of his crackers is both funny and sad. How satisfying is recovery if we choose food that would cause even a mouse to turn up his nose? How much should we sacrifice ourselves in order to save some calories?

In *Satisfaction and the Foods We Eat*, the author asks, "Is 'not bad' good enough?" And suggests, "No amount of what you don't want will fill you up."[2]

You may get some pleasure out of being virtuous in your eating, but dissatisfaction with food will always backfire.

What is Normal Eating?

In her first therapy session, Charlotte was distressed, "I am so sick and tired of yo-yo dieting. I gain, I lose. I starve myself. Then I over-eat. I wish I could just learn to eat normally. But I don't even know what normal eating is! What does that actually mean?"

Many people consider it normal—business as usual—to anxiously monitor their weight every day, worry about their amount of exercise, obsess about whether to eat dessert, and earnestly work to be good dieters. They equate self-esteem with how well they're controlling their food. But is a lifetime of guilt about food and weight really normal? Is constantly scrutinizing our food, calories, and size really how we want to live our whole life? Is our physical appearance the only way we want to measure our achievement in the world? Do we want to define ourselves as successful based on the ability to *control* ourselves, rather than cultivating our ability to *express* ourselves?

Disordered Eating Patterns: Obstacles to Normal Eating

Healing eating disorders is not only about resolving underlying emotional issues. It is also about concretely improving one's relationship with food—moving from chaotic eating to contented eating. People with disordered eating tend to follow some common patterns:

- Not eating structured meals.
- Snacking/grazing throughout the day.
- Only eating salad.
- Eliminating certain food groups, such as protein or fat or carbs.
- Drinking coffee or diet soda rather than eating food.
- Undereating during the day, only to binge at night.
- Eating only sugary foods or salty foods or alternating sugar/salt.
- Using gum, candy, vitamins, antacids, diet teas, bran, or alcohol as a substitute for food.

Over the years, my clients have provided many examples of what is *not* normal eating. A very common behavior is eating very rapidly. Clients have described "inhaling" their food, "wolfing it down," or as one imaginative girl described, "I don't chew; I gargle my food."

Lilly complains that her eating was "good" all day but she "ruined" it with cookies after dinner. Her guilt causes her to keep on bingeing.

Eliza feels guilty for cheating on her diet because she never counted the calories of the milk she added to her frequent daily coffees.

Stacey goes to a party, overeats, feels guilty, and then starves herself the next day.

Kathryn doesn't want to go to the movies with friends because she didn't exercise for a couple of days and feels "too fat."

Thomas binges on a pint of ice cream and makes himself throw up.

Chuck chooses only foods that are low-fat and low-calorie, no matter what he is really hungry for.

Lilly, Eliza, Stacey, Kathryn, Thomas, and Chuck feel inadequate and unhappy with themselves which affects their mood, their self-esteem, and fuels the critical voice in their heads which, in turn, leads to even more chaotic eating.

Here's what normal, healthy eating could look like for each of them:

Lilly has cookies after dinner and enjoys them, knowing that normal people eat cookies sometimes and they will not ruin her life.

Eliza realizes picking on herself for little transgressions, like guilt over the milk in her coffee, never helps. In fact, it often backfires, causing her to throw in the towel and eat everything in sight.

Stacey goes to a party, overeats, realizes she doesn't like

feeling overstuffed, and the next day goes back to eating when she is hungry.

Kathryn recognizes she will feel isolated and deprived if she doesn't socialize with her friends, decides to go to the movies, and promises herself she will return to exercising when she has the time and energy.

Thomas stops eating the ice cream when he feels full, knowing he can have it again whenever he wishes. Or Thomas binges on a pint of ice cream and does *not* make himself throw up. Bingeing without purging is a healthier option than bulimia, and it represents progress for the bulimic.

Chuck decides that restricting himself has only made his food problem worse. He decides to try choosing from a wider variety of foods.

Lilly, Eliza, Stacey, Kathryn, Thomas, and Chuck recognize that they are human, that sometimes they overeat or underexercise, and that life (and eating) is generally not perfect. They move on from there, living their day to the fullest, accepting their imperfections.

Developing Normal Eating

We all eat on a continuum from erratic, thoughtless, and unconscious on one end to hypervigilant, super-aware, and orthorexic on the other hand. Orthorexia refers to an obsession with healthy eating characterized by rigidly fixating on eating the perfect diet. Food journalist Mark Bittman has introduced the idea of striving to eat in the middle of the spectrum, to become a "flexitarian." According to Bittman, a flexitarian is a moderate and conscious eater.[3]

What are these rules to normal eating? There are none, because no one set of rules applies to everyone. Developing normal eating is an individual process based on your appetite, weight, metabolism, lifestyle, and activity level. And what's normal for you may even change from day to day!

Sometimes I want three meals a day and snacks, some days I want all my food to be breakfast food, sometimes I want a midnight snack, sometimes I want a ton of salad, sometimes I want a juicy hamburger with lots of ketchup. *The key to normal eating is tuning in to what you want to eat when you are hungry for it and stop eating when you are full.*

Normal eaters *generally*:

1. Eat meals.
2. Eat meals that have a beginning, middle, and end.
3. Eat balanced meals that include protein, carbohydrates, vegetables and/or fruits, some healthy fat.
4. Eat when they are hungry.
5. Eat what they really like without labeling food as good or bad.
6. Choose foods that will satisfy them.
7. Eat slowly, tasting and relishing what they're eating. And they chew!
8. Stop eating when they feel full and gratified.
9. Have snacks when hungry. Snacks, like meals, have a beginning, middle, and end.
10. Have certain personal guidelines to regulate their food intake—some structure, some shut-off valve that signals you are getting full and have had enough for now.
11. Face feelings directly, rather than detouring them through overeating or undue restriction. Sometimes they may over- or undereat because of stress, and sometimes they overeat just because the food tastes great.
12. Express their emotions directly, rather than stuffing food.
13. Forgive themselves if they overeat, undereat, or gain a couple of pounds. They take these fluctuations in stride as part of the normal ebb and flow of life.

14. Are flexible and not overly rigid if they cannot get exactly the food they want.
15. Consider food to be an important aspect of life but do not obsess or worry excessively about it. The recognize food is not the only love relationship in the world!
16. Enjoy food as one of the pleasures of life.

Nobody with an eating disorder becomes a normal eater overnight. But you can begin by making slow changes by following the above steps. If you accept that progress—not perfection—is your goal, you will come to live in better harmony with your body and your eating. Some wise person once said, "Anything worth doing, is worth doing *imperfectly*."

The End of Overeating

"It's not your fault!" states Dr. David Kessler in *The End of Overeating: Taking Control of the Insatiable American Appetite*. "America, has become a food fun house . . . a carnival of delicious, fatty, salty, sugary accessible and cheap delights. And how could you expect to go to the carnival and not want to go on the rides?"[4]

Dr. Kessler, a former commissioner of the U.S. Food and Drug Administration and former dean of Yale Medical School, analyzes the American diet and discovers how it contributes to America's struggle with overeating. He points out that foods laden with sugar, fat, and salt are taking our brains hostage! Fat + sugar + salt is so intensely appealing to the pleasure center in our brains that we are compelled to overeat, regardless of whether we are hungry!

Our brain's pleasure center helps us relax and reduce stress. Eating fat + sugar + salt is entertainment for our brains. No wonder the potato chip company dares us to eat just one!

Rather than blaming us for our lack of willpower, Dr. Kessler explains that the multi-billion dollar food industry has been remarkably successful in designing foods that seduce us and stimulate us to overeat.

An influential food executive explains to Kessler that the industry produces food with *excess* sugar, salt, and fat for the express purpose of appealing to the consumer to eat more and thus buy more. A vicious cycle gets created: be tempted > eat > buy food > be tempted > eat > buy more food.

No wonder Americans have gotten significantly fatter in recent years than ever before. With the growth in the number of restaurants, larger portions served, easily available take-out foods, warehouse supermarkets, all-night delis, and enticing television ads, food is calling to us loud and clear, 24 hours a day.

I came to realize the bounty of food in the United States and the unending availability of a wide variety of snacks when I visited Castro's Cuba. There I watched Cuban people line up at little hole-in-the-wall shops to purchase one single egg. That was all their ration books entitled them to. When I returned to the United States, I registered more fully the unlimited variety of cookies, cakes, muffins, candies, pastries, and even something as basic as endless varieties of yogurt for sale. A blessing, to be sure, but sometimes a curse.

Dr. Kessler explains how our everyday foods tempt us intensely without our full awareness. Many designer coffee concoctions are high in sugar and fat. Pizza is made with crusts of fat and salt with heavy cheese on top. Donuts are fat and sugar; salad dressings contain fat, salt, and sugar; chocolate chip cookies are full of fat, salt, and sugar. And some cereals stimulate the appetite with four or five combinations of sugar: brown sugar, fructose, corn syrup, honey, table sugar, and molasses, all exciting the pleasure center in our brains to cry out for more.

Even the *diet* cereal from Nutrisystem, NutriFrosted Crunch Cereal, contains an astonishing array of five different sweeteners: high fructose corn syrup, evaporated cane juice, barley malt extract, sugar, and malt flavoring!

In addition to sugar, fat, and salt, Kessler notes three other variables that increase our urge to eat even when we're not hungry:

1.   Quantity. Give people two scoops of ice cream and they automatically tend to eat both; three scoops and they'll eat three.
2.   Concentration. The more fat, salt, or sugar that is added to food, the more irresistible it becomes.
3.   Variety. Foods that have multiple layers of flavors increase their enticement—cookies with salty peanut butter plus chocolate covering, cinnamon raisin bagels, sweet and sour Chinese food, sweet and salty caramel popcorn.

Breaking the craving for foods laden with fat, sugar, and salt can be challenging, but several remedies can help:

1.   Keep consciously aware of the temptation that sugar, salty, and fatty food exerts on human biochemistry. Habitual overeating is a biological challenge; it is not a character flaw.
2.   Choose foods that satisfy you. Protein and high-fiber foods help keep you satisfied the longest. Fruits and vegetables supply fiber, vitamins, and even some protein; fruit can satisfy the desire for something sweet. *When we satisfy our hunger with nutritious food, the yearning to overeat will diminish.*
3.   Get support. Be accountable to a group, friend, or therapist. Involving another person in the struggle helps sustain one's resolve.

Nutrition Knowledge

Americans have more food to eat than any other nation on Earth and more diets to keep us from enjoying it.
—Cindy Adams, *New York Post,* August 19, 2011

Increasing our knowledge of nutrition offers another line of defense against disordered eating patterns and mindless eating.

Fat: Understanding Good and Bad Fats

The slogans "a moment on the lips, an inch on the hips" and "you are what you eat" cause people to wonder if food with fat will automatically get transplanted to their thighs! And so they eliminate all fats from their diet, not realizing that dietary fat is different from body fat.

Not all fats are created equal. Three categories of dietary fat have varying degrees of healthiness: unsaturated, saturated, and trans fats.

1. Unsaturated fats are healthy fats. These include monounsaturated and polyunsaturated fats. Monounsaturated fats raise the body's good cholesterol levels (HDL) and lower unhealthy cholesterol (LDL). Canola oil, olive oil, peanut oil, nuts, seeds, and avocados are good sources of monounsaturated fats.[5]

Polyunsaturated fats are also found in nuts, seeds, and vegetable oils, such as corn and safflower oil. Fatty fish, such as albacore tuna, salmon, sardines, and mackerel, also contains healthy polyunsaturated fats. The omega-3 and omega-6 oils contained in these foods are called essential fatty acids because our bodies must have them but do not produce them. We need to get them from food, just like vitamins. Omega-3s lower triglycerides and blood pressure, fight inflammation, and help blood clotting.

2. Saturated fats are unhealthy in large amounts. Saturated fat is found in animal foods such as meat and dairy products. In large amounts, saturated fat increases total cholesterol and LDL and may increase the risk of type 2 diabetes. Some plant foods, such as palm and coconut oil, also have saturated fat. Saturated fat carries the same risks whether derived from an animal or vegetable source.

3. Trans fats are liquid vegetable oils that have been heavily processed to stay solid at room temperature. They are found in many processed and fried foods. Trans fats are known to increase total

cholesterol and LDL (bad) cholesterol and lower HDL, the good cholesterol. Trans fats are also associated with a higher risk of type 2 diabetes, heart disease, and other serious health issues.

If the food label contains the words hydrogenated, partially hydrogenated, or shortening, this means the food contains trans fats and should be avoided or eaten in limited amounts.

According to the 2010 Dietary Guidelines for Americans, adults should get 20 percent to 35 percent of their calories from fat and no more than 10 percent of total calories from saturated fat.

Learning the difference between healthy and unhealthy fats is important so you don't deprive your body of the benefits of the healthy ones. Healthy fats are essential for brain function. The brain is made up of 60 percent fat. Diets that are too low in fat have been linked to Alzheimer's disease, memory loss, and dementia. Healthy fats also prevent and reduce symptoms of depression. Most people are not aware that very low cholesterol levels have been implicated in depression and even suicide. Healthy fats keep your skin and hair healthy. Healthy fats keep your blood sugar stable which is vital for weight loss and maintenance. They also improve insulin sensitivity which helps prevent and treat type 2 diabetes. Healthy fats also increase the body's ability to absorb fat-soluble vitamins, such as vitamin A and vitamin E. You also need healthy fats to reduce the risk of heart disease, stroke, and cancer, ease arthritis, joint pain, and inflammatory skin conditions, and support a healthy pregnancy.

Nutritional Support

Many psychotherapists in the field of eating disorders work with other healthcare professionals to leave no stone unturned to help their patients get better. A primary care physician, a psychiatrist if medication is needed, and a nutritionist can all be part of the professional team. If necessary, I will refer a psychotherapy patient to

Laura Shammah, a nutritionist and registered dietician, for extra nutritional support. For example, a patient with anorexia needs her calories and weight monitored; patients with diabetes, gestational diabetes, heart disease, or nutritional needs after chemotherapy have special dietary requirements that can benefit from professional advice.

The nutrition articles below were contributed by Laura Shammah, MS, RD.

Eat Breakfast!

For years, nutritionists have stated that breakfast is the most important meal of the day. Breakfast is so crucial because it provides that initial burst of energy needed after a good night's sleep and helps you perform better all day. By providing your brain with enough fuel to work properly, breakfast improves your concentration, coordination and enhances your mood. Also, eating breakfast increases the rate at which you burn calories so you have more energy and are less hungry.

Without breakfast, your body does not function optimally. Without the extra energy that breakfast provides, people often feel lethargic and turn to excess caffeine to get them through the day.

Studies show that people who skip breakfast tend to compensate by eating those calories later in the day, often choosing unhealthy, high-fat and high-calorie foods making weight control more difficult. This is particularly detrimental if those foods and snacks are low in fiber, vitamins and minerals but high in fat and salt.

Several studies suggest that people tend to accumulate more body fat when they eat fewer, larger meals than when they eat the same number of calories in smaller, more frequent meals.

Of course, not all breakfasts are created equal. Many Americans tend to start the day with pastries, high-calorie muffins and sugar-coated cereals. This is not supportive of your body; foods full of refined sugars offer calories without essential nutrients. High sugar foods and drinks may also cause your energy to soar briefly then abruptly fall, causing you to feel more drained and hungry a couple of hours later.

To avoid the sugar slump, choose whole grain breads and cereals and fresh fruits. These foods will give you longer-lasting energy. Healthy breakfasts might include:

- High fiber cereal or oatmeal with milk and fruit
- Yogurt and a piece of fruit
- English muffin toast with peanut butter and a glass of milk
- Pita with low fat cheese
- Cereal bar or granola bar and a glass of milk
- A shake or smoothie made with fruit and milk
- Low fat waffles with fruit and yogurt
- An omelet with a variety of vegetables
- Whole wheat bread

A healthy breakfast provides a significant proportion of the day's total nutrient intake and offers the opportunity to eat foods fortified with nutrients such as folate, iron, B vitamins and fiber.

It is important for parents to educate their children about the value of breakfast and its role in maintaining good health and preventing obesity. Studies have found that children who eat breakfast are better able to pay attention and are more focused on learning while those children who do not eat breakfast or grab a donut on the way to school are more likely to make poor food choices for the rest of the day.

Many teenage girls mistakenly believe that skipping breakfast is a perfectly logical way to cut down on calories and lose weight and need to be taught the health and energy benefits of having that first meal of the day.

Eating breakfast each morning starts your day out right. Make sure it's healthy, full of fiber and vitamins and your body will support you with energy and the ability to focus.

The Abundant Benefits of Fiber

When reading about nutrition and good health, one word pops up more than any other—fiber. Nutritionists have found that consuming fiber each day has abundant health benefits.

There are two types of fiber: soluble and insoluble. *Soluble* fiber dissolves in water and is found in oat bran, dried beans and peas, nuts, barley, flax seed, oranges, apples and carrots. Soluble fiber helps to regulate the flow of waste through the digestive tract.

Insoluble fiber cannot be dissolved in water, meaning that your body cannot digest it. Good sources of insoluble fiber include dark green leafy vegetables, fruit skins, root vegetable skins and wheat bran. This fiber is important because it helps keep your colon healthy.

Most nutritionists recommend 25 to 40 grams of fiber every day. Unfortunately, most people only consume 8 to 15 grams per day. To increase fiber in the diet, add whole-grain breads, high fiber cereals, whole wheat pasta, brown rice, dried beans, peas, lentils, nuts, fruits, and vegetables. An apple and almonds make a perfect snack.

Eating a fiber rich diet improves health significantly by improving bowel function, lowering cholesterol, reducing one's risk of colon and breast cancer. Fiber helps people with diabetes by reducing the amount of insulin released by the pancreas. It also lowers triglycerides, a type of fat found in the blood. Although the body uses triglycerides for energy, high triglycerides can raise your risk of heart disease.

Eating fiber can also help lose weight by acting as an appetite suppressant. Once ingested, soluble fiber absorbs water and swells. This provides you with a feeling of fullness and curbs your appetite. It also helps reduce blood sugar swings, by steadily releasing sugar into the bloodstream, reducing hunger pangs, headaches, and fatigue caused by a rapid drop in blood sugar.

Foods that are rich in fiber generally take longer to chew which automatically slows down the speed of consumption. Fiber helps to reduce the absorption of fat, and eating more fiber will help trigger the "satisfaction response" and signaling the "I'm full" message.

Foods that are high in fiber include:

- Beans: baked, kidney, dried, lima, garbanzo, pinto and black
- Whole wheat and other whole-grain products: rye, oats, buckwheat and bran cereals
- Dried fruits: figs, apricots and dates
- Other fruits: raspberries, blackberries, strawberries, cherries, bananas, plums, apples and pears.
- Vegetables: corn, broccoli, spinach, beet greens, kale, collards, Swiss chard, carrots, Brussels sprouts and turnip greens
- Nuts and seeds: especially almonds, Brazil nuts, peanuts, walnuts and flax seeds. The flax seed is one of nature's best health foods. It is rich in omega-3 fatty acids, soluble fiber, and protein. While nuts are high in fiber, they're also high in fat, so they should be eaten sparingly.

A healthy goal is to eat 40 grams of fiber each day.

Eat Right and Sustain Health

Researchers have found cholesterol deposits in the arteries of teens and young adults and even young children due to diets full of high fat, low fiber and fried foods.

We age along a continuum. We don't wake up one morning with wrinkles and gray hair. Aging is a process that begins in our early adult years. Osteoporosis and heart disease are caused by a lifetime of eating unhealthy foods—foods high in fat and low in nutritional value. That's why it is so important that we start early teaching our children to eat more nutrient-rich foods.

Foods that are low in fiber and high in fat, such as burgers and fries, promote constipation and can cause diverticulitis, a painful condition of the colon that afflicts half of all Americans over the age of 60. Add an inactive lifestyle and stress, and you will age early and faster.

The alternate scenario is much more beneficial. Eating calcium-rich foods, lots of fruits, vegetables, lean meats and fiber from whole grains will help keep your bowel movements regular and the antioxidants from fruits and vegetables will help prevent cancer.

Eating vegetables, fruits and whole grains will sustain and strengthen our bodies, our bones and our hearts.

It's never too late to begin eating a healthy, high fiber diet. It will slow the aging process and make you feel stronger and more vigorous.

Water, Water Everywhere: But Are We Drinking It?
Water helps keep your muscles and skin toned, assists in weight loss, transports oxygen and nutrients to cells, eliminates toxins and wastes from the body, and regulates body temperature. Drinking refreshing, clean water plays a major role in reducing the risk of certain diseases. Water is the most neglected nutrient in your diet, but one of the most vital.

Most people need six to eight cups a day. You will know if you are drinking enough if your urine is transparent or almost clear.

Here are a few ways to help you increase your water consumption:

1. Instead of caffeine and alcohol, drink water. Caffeine and alcohol act as diuretics and cause the body to lose water.
2. Throughout the day, have water constantly available; keep a water bottle on your desk; carry a bottle of water with you when you are on the go.
3. Create a daily schedule; drink a glass after breakfast, one before lunch, with each snack.
4. Ask for a glass of water with your coffee or tea in cafes.
5. Eat a selection of fruit and vegetables as these have high water

content and will contribute to your daily water intake.

6. If you do not like water, drink seltzer. Just make sure it is sodium-free.

Two-thirds of your body weight is water, so keep well hydrated. Your metabolism will appreciate it!

Prevent the Blood Sugar Roller Coaster: Keeping Energy Stable
Everyone can benefit from keeping their blood sugar low and stable, and it is possible to do that with the foods you eat and the frequency in which you eat them. Of course, you should consult a doctor before any drastic diet changes, and if you are diabetic, stay in frequent touch with your doctor to monitor the need for any insulin adjustments. Many people have grown up with the idea that it's best to eat three square meals a day. But going too many hours without eating causes your sugar levels to go up and down like a roller coaster. Ultimately, you will be much more satisfied, eat less, and maintain a stable blood sugar level throughout the day if you eat smaller meals every two to three hours, for a total of about six meals a day.

The content of those meals does matter. The better quality of foods you eat, the more satisfied you'll feel between meals. Every meal should be a balance of two primary components: lean protein and carbohydrates.

First, protein will help keep you from getting hungry between meals, and the better quality of protein, the better it is for you. Good choices of protein include lean chicken, turkey or beef, low fat cheeses, cottage cheese and eggs. Eggs have a reputation for being unhealthy, but they are actually a very healthy option. The fat in eggs is the kind your body needs; just eat them in moderation. Eating one whole egg plus two or three egg whites to provide the benefits of protein without the extra fat.

Balancing out the protein with good-quality carbohydrates will give you energy. Carbs have gotten a bad rap over the last few years, but there are healthy carbs and not healthy carbs. Carbs that are basically sugar have no nutritional value. Carbs such as whole grains, fruits and vegetables offer you energy while keeping your blood sugar from spiking. Bread should have at least three grams of fiber per slice. Choose brown rice and whole wheat pasta. In fact, the first ingredient of your bread or pasta should include the word "whole." Eat as many vegetables as you want with at least two of your meals each day, and fruit with one or two meals as well.

With the combination of high quality protein and whole grain carbohydrates eaten in small quantities every few hours, you will not only keep your metabolism burning evenly, but you'll also keep your blood sugar right where it should be, without the spikes or resulting crashes. You'll feel more energy and maybe even see an improvement in your mood.

Managing Food Cravings: A Nutritionist's Perspective

How many times has this happened to you? After a great start at eating healthy in an attempt to lose weight, the cookies begin to call you. Pretty soon, half the box is gone, along with your latest attempts at weight management.

Many people think that the only way to lose weight and keep it off is by eliminating high-fat, high-calorie foods entirely. Many weight control programs today call these foods "addictive" and recommend giving them up forever. While you think giving up such foods may help you gain better control over your eating, the truth is you are actually giving up control. Your craving for the foods you love will remain and may even become stronger. To adopt a healthy eating plan that includes the foods you crave, try these tips:

Eat at least three well-balanced meals a day. Even if you're trying to lose weight, don't skip meals. You'll only be hungrier for the next one, and cravings between meals can become overwhelming.

Give up guilt. Believing you have cheated on your diet and completely ruined your chances of succeeding produces guilt and feelings of failure. Give yourself permission to eat favorite foods in moderation and without guilt.

Accept food cravings as a normal part of living in a food-oriented society. Almost everyone experiences food cravings, regardless of whether they struggle with their weight. The more you understand your cravings, the better you can manage them. While you cannot control the fact that cravings occur, you can control your reaction.

Think "management" instead of "control." "Control" implies an adversarial relationship with food; it's generally a constant struggle to maintain control. "Management" is much easier. When we manage something, we work in partnership with it to achieve our desired results.

Look at cravings as suggestions to eat, not commands to over-indulge. Overeating does not have to be an automatic response to a craving. When a craving begins, determine how you want to deal with it. It is truly up to you. You have choices.

Believe that cravings will pass. A craving is similar to an ocean wave. It grows in intensity, peaks, and then subsides whether or not you jump into it. Picture yourself as a surfer who is trying to "ride the wave," instead of being wiped out by it. The more you practice riding the wave, the easier it will become.

Disarm your cravings with the five Ds:

• Delay at least 10 minutes before you eat so that your action is conscious, not impulsive.

• Distract yourself by engaging in an activity that requires concentration.

• Distance yourself from the food.

• Determine how important it really is for you to eat the craved food and how much you really want it.

• Decide what amount is reasonable and appropriate, eat it slowly and enjoy!

Stop labeling foods as bad, illegal or forbidden. It's not the food itself that's the problem, but the quantities you consume and how often you consume them. You can eat whatever you want—even if it is high in fat, calories or sugar—but to reach your goals, you may not be able to eat all of everything you want every time you want it.

Aim for moderation instead of abstinence. Avoiding foods you fear only reinforces the fear. Practice enjoying reasonable amounts of favorite high-fat or high-calorie foods. You may be happier and better able to stay with a well-balanced plan for healthy living.

Exercise regularly. Just as it is important to successfully manage your weight, exercise is key to managing food cravings. In addition to burning calories, regular exercise may bring relief from tension due to anxieties about food cravings. It is also another way to delay, distance, and distract yourself from food.

Enjoying Your Food

Punishment, restriction, and guilt are more familiar concepts for emotional eaters than actually enjoying their food. However, reclaiming the real pleasure of eating, meals, food, and variety is key to a full and fruitful recovery.

Declaring peace with emotional eating involves enjoying your food. Food, glorious food!

Bon appétit!	(French)
Buen provecho!	(Spanish)
Buon appetito!	(Italian)
Kali orexi!	(Greek)
Guten Appetit!	(German)
Goede eetlust!	(Dutch)
Bom apetite!	(Portuguese)
Hyvä ruokahalu!	(Finnish)
Dobry apetyt!	(Polish)
B'tayavon!	(Hebrew)

1   William N. Davis, *The Renfrew Perspective* (Renfrew Center Foundation).

2   Karin Kratina, "Satisfaction and the Foods We Eat," *The Journal of Health at Every Size,* Summer 2006, vol. 20, number 2, 75–81.

3   Mark Bittman, "Healthy, Meet Delicious," *New York Times,* April 24, 2013.

4   David Kessler, *The End of Overeating: Taking Control of the Insatiable American Appetite* (Rodale, 2010).
    Pandora's Lunchbox, by Melanie Warner (Scribner, 2013), critiques how the processed food industry seduces the American public. Processed foods, laden with salt, sugar, fat, and chemicals, accounts for 70 percent of the calories Americans consume annually. She reveals the 105 ingredients in the popular, and allegedly healthy, Subway Sweet Onion Teriyaki sandwich. The chicken alone contains: potassium chloride, maltodextrin, autolyzed yeast extract, gum arabic, soy protein concentrate, and sodium phosphates. The bread contains: ammonium sulfate, azodicarbonamide, potassium iodate, sodium stearoyl lactylate.
    Salt Sugar Fat: How the Food Giants Hooked Us, by *New York Times* reporter Michael Moss (Random House, 2013), exposes the processed food industry for the "deliberate and calculating" effort they make to discover the physiological "bliss point" which will hook consumers to eat/buy/eat/buy more. He claims corporate scientists consciously manipulate processed food "to make people feel hungrier." He likens the food industry to the tobacco industry, to be viewed as a "public health menace."

5   To help remember which cholesterol is good and which is bad: *H*DL (Healthy) and *L*DL (Lousy).

Epilogue. Life after Eating Disorders

As we finish the meal we have shared together of *Lasagna for Lunch*, I am reminded of the poem written by Kayla at the conclusion of her therapy for binge eating disorder.

> *The Guided Tour*
> Kayla
>
> *The guided tour is over.*
> *Most of all my fears are gone.*
> *The park is closing*
> *I'll find my way out alone*
>
> *And with every turn I'll use the lessons I have learned.*

The lessons we have learned are summarized in my "recipe for recovery" for emotional eating. Only two of the ingredients have to do with food! These lessons have to do with your ability to:

- Eat when you are hungry and stop when you are full.
- View food as a friend and ally, something to be enjoyed and not feared.
- Identify feelings—anger, sadness, resentment, disappointment, sexuality, envy—without detouring them through food.

- Express your feelings directly.
- Learn to grieve, cry, and mourn the losses in your life.
- Tolerate the discomfort of anxiety, loneliness, fear, and boredom, knowing that it will pass whether or not you eat over it.
- Judge yourself and your feelings with compassion and understanding, rather than harsh condemnation.
- Enjoy your sexuality and communicate with a partner without shame.
- Appreciate and accept your body, no matter what your current size.
- Develop humor about your human foibles, knowing that we are "all more human than not."
- Develop relationships with others in which you feel safe enough to be your real and genuine self.
- Comfort and soothe yourself in ways other than food.
- Anything worth doing is worth doing imperfectly. Be uniquely you.
- Cultivate your hunger for emotional truth, connection, and love.

As Oscar Wilde said, "Be yourself; everyone else is already taken."

The experience of a fruitful therapy is expressed so touchingly in this excerpt from a poem by Meredith. May every reader declare peace with emotional eating and learn to claim the beauty of life.

Locked Out with No Key
Meredith

Locked out with no key
To get inside
No bell, no doorman
All options I tried.

I knocked and banged
Feeling so alone and forsaken
I must get inside to stabilize
My inner world that was so shaken.

My heart ached with pain
I thought I am absurd
But finally by someone
My plea was heard.

The door was opened
Opened very wide
With much trepidation in my steps
I slowly walked inside.

I questioned and doubted
Is this where I belong?
I heard many unwanted voices
But kept myself strong.

And I'm still here now
Because this is what I choose to do
Today I am witness
That my inkling was true.

The door was locked
You gave me the key
Look at me now
For yourself you'll see.

I've gone through many doors
Learned to feel and to react

Traveling with me on my journey
Has made a tremendous impact.

You stood by me through these trying times
And still do so today
I have passion and experience life
In a whole new way.

Also available:

French Toast for Breakfast:
Declaring Peace with Emotional Eating

French Toast has been described as a "warm and compassionate guide to understand the emotions that underlie eating disorders. Filled with practical exercises, dialogues from actual therapy session, an in-depth comparison of treatment options, and a look at relapse—how to prevent it and what to do if it occurs. It also includes a unique questionnaire to help readers determine which path to peace is best for them."

Praise for *French Toast:*

"A wise and wonderful, sensitive and sane contribution. Beautifully written."
—Judy Rusky Rabinor, Ph.D.

"*French Toast for Breakfast* expresses everything you wish your therapist had told you about how to resolve your eating problems. 99% of therapists don't deal with the depth that Mary Anne Cohen does. Terrific examples, awesome."
—Joanne Gerr, LCSW

"Clearly and effectively describes the intimate connection between eating disorders and the emotional pain that causes them. Transcripts of therapy sessions take readers directly into the treatment room and make them part of the healing process. This book will appeal to a wide audience because it demystifies the process of psychotherapy."
—Janet David, Ph.D.

"Expertly and gently guides the reader to a personal understanding of emotional eating and offers strategies for change and hope for peace."
—Edward Spauster, Ph.D.

Order form on following page.

ORDER FORM

Please send me
French Toast for Breakfast: Declaring Peace with Emotional Eating

Each copy: $14.95 + $3 shipping and handling
New Yorkers please add 8.25 % tax

Name:_____

Address:_____

City, State, Zip:_____

Phone:_____

e-mail:_____

Please send check or money order to:

Mary Anne Cohen
490 Third Street
Brooklyn New York 11215
718-788-6986
www.EmotionalEating.Org